S0-BWZ-031

IRONWOMEN NEVER RUST

Making Memories
While Managing Menopause

By Emily G. Bruno, R.N.C., M.S.N

Emily G. Bruno

To Ellen,
We are loving being
neighbors with ya'll!!
Love,
Emily
July '05

Westview
Publishing, Inc.
Nashville, Tennessee

© 2003 by Emily G. Bruno

All rights reserved, including the right to reproduce this book or any part thereof in any form whether in print, electronic format or any other media. Reviewers may use brief excerpts with the permission of the author or publisher.

First Edition

ISBN 0-9744322-7-X

Library of Congress Control Number: 2003115448

Printed in the United States of America

Edited by Susan G. Brown

Cover Design by Hugh Daniel

Layout, cover design and other pre-press by Westview Publishing, Inc.

Westview Publishing, Inc.
8120 Sawyer Brown Road, Ste. 107
Nashville, TN 37221
(615) 646-6131
http://www.westviewpublishing.com

This book is dedicated with love to the most influential men in my life: my father, whose example has steered me, my two brothers Sam and Bim, whose ages bracketed mine and whose treatment of me kept me from taking myself too seriously, my three sons John, Keith, and Will, whose lives have taught me the many facets of caring, and, most importantly, my husband Johnny, whose quiet support has never failed me. I am the woman I am today in large measure because of my life with them.

"As both a physician and a runner, I deeply appreciate the vital message contained in Emily Bruno's book, linking regular exercise to a life of increased health and contentment for women, especially in their mature years. She proves that it's never too late to start."

Byron Haitas, M.D.
Cardiovascular Medicine
Frist Cardiology, PLLC,
Nashville, Tennessee

"Bruno takes us on her extraordinary journeys of accomplishments and pain. Yet her message is for all women; take the first step, be determined, and all of us can have extraordinary journeys. A wonderful read!"

Pam Hutcherson
Women's Health Nurse, Author
and Business Owner

CONTENTS

–Donating blood
–More on HRT and herbals

2001
Powerman Alabama Duathlon - Birmingham,
Alabama *(6.2 mile run, 36 mile bike, 3.1 mile run)*
Lion's Journey for Sight Biathlon - Murfreesboro,
Tennessee *(6.2 mile run, 26.4 mile bike)*
Tennessee State Championship Triathlon -
Chattanooga, Tennessee *(0.9 mile swim, 25 mile
bike, 6.2 mile run)*
Vineman Half Ironman Triathlon - Guerneville,
California *(1.2 mile swim, 56 mile bike, 13.2 mile
run)*
–More on mountain biking and hiking
–Speed work - should I run on a track?
–Osteoarthritis
National Championship Olympic-Distance Triathlon
- Coeur d'Alene, Idaho *(0.9 mile swim, 25 mile bike,
6.2 mile run)*
–Friendships through sport
World Championship Short Course Duathlon -
Rimini, Italy *(6.2 mile run, 25 mile bike, 3.1 mile
run)*
Race for the Cure 5K - Nashville, Tennessee *(3.1 mile
run)*
–New studies on benefits and risks of HRT

Afterword
World Championship Long Course Duathlon - Weyer,
Austria *(8.4 mile run, 48 mile bike, 4.2 mile run)*
World Championship Ironman Triathlon - Kona,
Hawaii *(2.4 mile swim, 112 mile bike, 26.2 mile
run)*

World Championship Short Course Triathlon - Cancun, Mexico *(0.9 mile swim, 25 mile bike, 6.2 mile run)*

ACKNOWLEDGMENTS

I wish to thank sincerely all the friends, family members, and colleagues who provided valid suggestions and great encouragement in the creation of this book.

Special gratitude goes to my sister, Susan G. Brown for her wonderful expertise in editing.

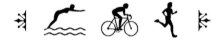

PREFACE

From ballerinas to barrel riders

And the beautiful princess married the handsome prince, and it came to pass that she bore him many children, and she fed them and kept their house and made it a home, and she was honored for this (mainly on Mothers' Day - well, most Mothers' Days). And as time passed her children grew, her husband's business prospered and required important commitments. Finally, as her children stood tall and left their nest, it seemed that the culmination of her earnest efforts had arrived. Instead, a melancholy prevailed as she saw her life's mission seemingly reach a conclusion just as her husband's life appeared most productive. Her social contacts seemed almost superficial, but they helped to allay the uneasiness which arrived with the first gray strands of hair and the flushing and night sweats that accompanied her loss of fertility.

Goodness, where's the happily-ever-after part? It is amazing how frequently this hyperbole recreates itself to some degree in the traditional family or even the family modified for today's increased financial needs. There can be an alienation from the vibrancy which defines so much of one's early life. While this pattern is not unique to women, it certainly traces the course of a woman's life more reliably than that of a man.

Any number of mechanisms could be devised to cope with or counter this pattern of emptiness or loss of self-esteem that can come from fulfilling a seemingly lifelong responsibility well before the end of one's life. Some of our friends and my patients have chosen to train for a ministry in organized religion. Volunteer

11

organizations are filled with productive and committed workers who come from these ranks. New companies are starting up with women at the helm who are beginning a new life for themselves after a life of service to their families.

The second half of the twentieth century was a remarkable period in the history of civilization. Trains gave way to planes in transportation, infant mortality plummeted in developed countries, infections and diseases that once carried a death sentence became eminently treatable, construction techniques allowed for increased population density and subsequent productivity while controlling to some degree the toll of crowding on the human psyche. Further, exploration into space, into the depths of our oceans and our planet, and exploration of the human organism and its mechanisms of function have been promoted in an unprecedented way. A more subtle change has taken place, however, that may have a more profound effect on the course of human development.

Women are hatching! Well, the avian metaphor may be a little steep, but in truth the ontological progression from a walled-in embryo to a bird of flight may not be so far afield. From the times of hunter-gatherer societies until well into the twentieth century, a woman required a male to be her voice. Even the most vociferous women, with carefully constructed ideas or plans, met daunting opposition were they to speak forthrightly in public without their "knight errant" to convey a symbol of power or presence. Dr. Elizabeth Alexander recounts in her biography <u>Notorious Woman</u> the passionate efforts of a nineteenth-century woman to claim her inheritance. It became a nationally-watched event and bordered on scandalous at times when she had to represent her case without the support of a male supervisor.

Though women's suffrage came early in the last

century, there was little dynamic for a change in their status before the Second World War brought women into the workplace in unprecedented numbers. That factor perhaps more than any other has been at the root of women's self-exploration. Being able to develop financial independence from the male led to issues of equal opportunity and an equal income for the same work done. The number of major business efforts started and run by women has increased dramatically. The percentage of women in medical and law school classes has skyrocketed. The world of women's athletics has changed no less dramatically.

For many years the athletic elegance of ballet was the only well-accepted outlet for athleticism in women. Incredible skill and training were packaged in such a way as to appear effortless, ethereal, and certainly without sweat. However, the ballerinas I have come to know are physically and psychologically tough; only the traditions of their sport/art form make them appear otherwise.

Until the last twenty to thirty years other female athletic involvement was limited to programs at all-girls secondary schools, colleges or universities, and following the end of school there was limited support for continuing any of the team sports which had been learned, with the possible exception of tennis. I well recall that at my public high school any female with real athletic potential squelched it for fear of social reprisal. At the same time, growing up in the sixties, I saw an enormous positive reinforcement for athletic participation by boys. Time passed before I realized the different forces at work on the women with whom I grew up. My first real awakening to this inequity occurred while I was still a college undergraduate. Males and females alike had a physical education requirement for one year, but girls were not allowed to walk across campus to their gym in shorts unless covered up with a raincoat. It is hard to imagine that this could have been possible in my lifetime but now I'm even more disturbed by how passively I accepted it.

Since the raincoats have been shed, women have lost little time in gaining ground. The explosion of women's organized athletics is tremendous, and their success in those sports is impressive. Women's basketball did not even exist as a sport in most schools thirty years ago, and now a sustainable professional league is active. Our whole nation was thrilled by our national women's soccer team several years ago, and its members became instant role models for girls all over this country. Watching the fluid movement of our women sprinters today reminds me how far they have come since my teenage years. Just as striking as these gains may be the way women have so successfully challenged the concept that they were not suited to endurance events. In the last twenty years men have managed to shave only a few minutes from the marathon world record, while women have reduced their record by twenty minutes, thus dramatically closing the gap between the sexes. This is not to praise the elite athlete to the exclusion of others, rather, to suggest that as women are freed to explore their physical limits, they gain another dimension of self awareness and self growth that adds resilience to their personalities. All of the positive qualities that "sport" has been said to imbue, such as endurance, determination, team work, and self reliance, are now available to women.

During more than twenty years of practice in sports medicine, I have watched the athlete emerge in young and old women alike. It may take the form of a high school student who deals calmly with a medical interview, demonstrating the inner confidence that also allows her to hit a clutch three-pointer at the end of a game or to reach a little deeper in the final stretch of a cross country race. Just as gratifying to see is the mid-fifties mother who has taken responsibility for her health and who comes in for treatment of a walking injury, determined to get back to the exercise routine that has given her a new perspective on life.

I believe that this record of my wife's experiences is proof positive of the confidence and inner strength that can be gained through athletic effort, determination, and perseverance.

John Bruno III, MD
Orthopaedic surgeon specializing
in Sportsmedicine

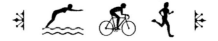

April 2000

"Afoot and light-hearted I take to the open road,
Healthy, free, the world before me,
The long brown path before me leading
wherever I choose."

Walt Whitman,
Song of the Open Road

The boys were mostly gone. One day I was dashing to and from sporting events, school plays, art shows, throwing hurried dinners on the table. Suddenly, I looked up and there was no one to cheer for, to defend, to absorb or dismiss my unsought words of wisdom. They come back from school, jobs, and travels periodically, for a few days or maybe weeks. When they do, they do not like to see change; they want their rooms to be just like they left them. They want us to be just the same, too.

But I have changed. Along with many of my responsibilities as a mother, my periods are gone, too. Mother Nature throws her energies into fertile young bodies. Like the new moon which grows a sliver at a time, with a gentler light than that of the dazzling sun, a whole new life was growing in me seemingly from nowhere; but like the new moon, the scaffolding for this development was there all along waiting for the necessary illumination to show its existence. Age appeared to be working for me - I was sneaking into menopause with the strands of gray hair at my temples camouflaged by the dishwater blonde. I was not abdicating my old life; I was discovering the freedoms which these changes were to bring. Of course, there were other roles to be filled and duties calling: ministering to friends whose spouses had left them for younger lovers, cooking and supporting those ravaged by old age or disease, working to pay our monthly bills. But my mother's words rang loud and clear: "There will always be beds to make." I refused to sit around and wait for things to happen to me; I would launch out and move on. I believe that all women can.

>─┤─◆〉─◦─O─◦─〈◆─┤─◄

We had an easy afternoon departure from Nashville, an easy evening arrival to and departure from Los Angeles. A silent, nonstop glide through the night to Sydney followed without a glitch. Nevertheless, flying this far is tough in the best of circumstances. I could not fathom how the missionary couple flying to Mongolia with their fretful four month old could make such a trip without going crazy. It may have something to do with the resilience of youth. Hundreds of bodies were hermetically sealed in a container which we never even saw from the outside; we did not know our collective color or our shape. For 14 hours we shared our five-person row with a pair, mother and son it seemed, she coughing a tubercular hack, he smelling like he'd not had a shower in a week. We never in all that time passed a word. I suppose we each had our own agenda and tried not to encroach on the other's space, either physically or verbally.

We continued to progress across the globe, crossing the international date line, but we somehow lost a day in the progression! Now better than halfway around the world, we found it hard simply to calculate what time it was anywhere. I was glad that I had brought an extra watch to keep set to Nashville time. When we whittled it down to five hours until we would arrive at our destination of Perth, Australia, that time and distance seemed trivial. Our internal clocks and our biorhythms were confused. The deep fatigue of wakefulness crept in, leaving us with that "blah" feeling. A fellow in front of us boarded the final leg of our trip, fresh from some connecting flight; well, I won't say fresh. He stood motionless, staring into space, ignoring the attendant who was trying to get his attention.

"Your ticket, please, sir." I don't think he was simple-minded; he must have had a bad case of jet-lag, too. Or, we decided, his wife wasn't with him, and he couldn't get it together.

All "day" a congregation of athletes streamed from various locations around the world into a widening river of fit bodies which would empty into Perth. Spotting a country logo on a backpack or jacket, I would try to figure out if this person was in my age group, sizing up where I stood in terms of competition. I knew deep down that any such assessment was foolish; champions emerge only on race day.

As we waited in the Sydney airport, a friendship was already developing with Mary, a potter from New York. The approach to our mutual destination was exciting, but a little nerve-racking. We talked about races we'd both done, how she had been training all winter (... the doubt that I hadn't done enough, or the right kind, began to nag me ....) In the haste of packing, she had left her biking shoes behind; no worry, her husband would FedEx them to her. Plans were already taking shape for riding, running, and swimming together. We kept eating - dishes I don't usually eat - expending only the energy required to walk through airports. Somehow my system must adjust to the food, the water, and the climate, with five days to go before the race. Would my bike make the trip without damage; would it make it at all?

The excitement and anticipation of an extended holiday began to collide with growing exhaustion. Eyeshades and ear plugs didn't compensate for our upright body position to allow real rest. The past weeks had been jammed with the usual last minute chores of leaving one's affairs in order, as well as continuing to train. Then throw in the stroke which Johnny's father suffered, his death, and our frenzied trip to the funeral five days before our departure; those were the makings of significant stress. I just hoped that I had not "caught" something from my sick-sounding seat mate as we flew over the ocean.

The bike made it to Perth! Like a surrogate mother, the pregnant 747 emptied its belly of dozens of bike boxes, a few with signs of rough handling. Mine was stripped of one of the two locks, but the gear inside was miraculously intact. Driving cautiously down the left side of the road, we entered a crisp, sunny climate alive with the chirps of tropical birds and waving palm trees. Perth reminded me of San Diego - with less traffic. After locating our hotel, we changed clothes and jogged down to the banks of the Swan River; sun exposure supposedly helps reset that internal clock.

An early dinner followed. Never had I thought I would eat kangaroo, but it was delicious. (I had heard that the animals are too plentiful, like the deer population in the South. Months later when the U.K. and European countries were besieged by Hoof and Mouth and Mad Cow Diseases, we heard that butchers were buying up this mild-flavored meat which is lean and wild-harvested, raised with no hormones.) Unlike some triathletes, I eat pretty much what I want, but basically a well-balanced diet; actually, most of my friends in the sport don't shun meat or desserts and enjoy all kinds of foods. The delightful scene at the cafe on the banks of the lovely Swan River eased our exhaustion from the trip. The lights played on the ripples, and Johnny framed make-believe photos as we sipped a fruity Australian chardonnay with our dinner.

We stopped to get ice cream cones for the walk back to the hotel. "So you're here for the race?" asked the Aussie as he dished them up. "I'd never swim in that river. The dirt runs down the hills into the river when it rains." This did nothing for my already shaky concern about the swim! News of sharks around the Sydney harbor had made national news. Rumor had it that this water was full of algae and jellyfish and that it was COLD; and one never knows if race directors will allow wetsuits until the morning of the race.

We collapsed into bed, exhausted, without exploring the intriguing city. Unfortunately, our circadian rhythms weren't fooled, and we were both bug-eyed in the early morning darkness. I was anxious to get out and see the run and bike courses. Several women in my age group, including Mary, the potter I had met the day before, were also up early in the hotel lobby, on the floor stretching. Plans included a run, breakfast, trip to a pool, and then biking the course. The idea sounded good to me. So we were off, and we spent all day getting to know one another, as well as the course. The final activity of the day was the ride. I decided to take a third loop on my bike through the hilly park overlooking the city when the others headed back to the hotel.

As I slowed down from climbing the last hill, my adrenaline about expended, I heard behind me "Oops, hey thar." The British accent surprised me as a woman whooshed up on my right. She had caught me on a hill, so I knew she was a strong cyclist. I heard the English/Australian accent right away (I hadn't yet learned to tell the difference), and figured she was local. "Are you from Nashville?" She'd seen the Music City logo on my shorts.

"Yes, are you from around here?"

"No, Tasmania." No horns, but a devil of a biker. Turned out she was the age group below me - I was relieved! We chatted as I huffed and puffed, determined to keep up with her. The Tasmanian team was five-strong; the American team had about 236 entrants. She shared with me the scuttlebutt that there were two very strong British women in my age group. We exchanged names and wished each other good luck.

What was this race that had me halfway around the globe, carting my bicycle, instead of sexy negligees? (Actually, I took one of those, too.) It was the Olympic-distance World Championship Triathlon for pros and age groups. Distances were 1.5 kilometers (0.9 mile) swim, 40 kilometers (25 miles) bike ride, and 10 kilometers (6.2 miles) run. Forty countries were represented, with more than 1200 competitors. Triathlon would be an Olympic sport for the first time this year, and, for some countries, this race was the qualifier for their Olympic team. At fifty-three, I was not the oldest competitor! There were men and women in their seventies competing right next to the young whippersnappers.

There would be thirty-one women in my age group. A national race in Saint Joseph, Missouri, the previous fall had been the qualifier for the top twelve athletes in the five-year age group increments. I placed fourth in that race, behind Ramona, Jean, and Evelyn. At mile six of the run portion of that race I had passed Rita; I could see the fifty-two (her age) marked on her right calf as I came from behind, and I had debated about how late in the race to make my move to go by her. Would she surge? Two tenths of a mile is a long way to sprint when you've already been working hard for more than two and a half hours. But I made the move, never looked back, and ran as hard as I could to the finish - not a pretty sight. With a grimace on my face, my "finish-line" picture was not a keeper.

Rita had been on the team when I went to the World Championship race at the Gold Coast, north of Brisbane in 1991, and I've seen her at races through the years. She's very strong and has done the Bicycle Race Across America (RAM). Chatting with her after that race in St. Joseph, I had apologized with a smile on my face for passing her so close to the finish line (Southern girls do that). She gave me a "you know you don't mean that" look and said, "Shut up," also smiling. She's a great spirit, the life-of-the-party sort; I have fond memories of us girls taking pictures on the beach in 1991 with naughty smiles and bare behinds. The truth is, she may have wanted revenge in Perth, but what is wonderful is that each of us had a sense of accomplishment to have made it to that level. There is a strong bond shared by women striving to stretch themselves through sports.

The opening ceremonies in Perth lacked the extravagant 50-foot-tall jellyfish, 1000 tap dancers, and liquid torch of the Olympics, but pleased the crowd in an intimate way. All the teams and lots of onlookers were entertained by an Aussie choral group and Aboriginal dancers singing and moving to the soulful sounds of a didgeridoo, followed by fireworks and the gracious words of welcome by the Minister of Tourism. He reported that more than 50,000 spectators were expected to be there "for the party" on Sunday. We were under a huge tent next to the transition area on the river banks. Unfortunately, it was quite windy with rain squalls periodically pounding, adding drama to the setting. The South African team started a "wave" which spread enthusiastically through the tent.

>─┼─◆>──O──<◆─┼─<

This trip was not the beginning of the story, of course. More than thirty years ago, after playing college football, Johnny had started running to shed weight, back when a person running down the street was assumed to be an escapee from prison or possibly a mental hospital. We were dating, and he would run from the college campus to my home, only about three miles. Mom would cook a large breakfast of eggs, bacon, and toast, after making certain that he was not going to die after such an ordeal. In a few years he started doing triathlons, and I served as his personal support team on more than one occasion. I would follow him around in the car, a child or two along for the ride, filling his water bottle, checking the map to make certain that he hadn't made a wrong turn and gotten lost (which happened to more than one competitor), and then hold up a towel while he changed into his running clothes. Now it is illegal to have anyone unofficial provide support. I began to suspect that it might be more fun out there participating, too, but I kept those thoughts to myself for a while. I held the few women competitors of those days on a pedestal. One might say that Johnny planted the seed and encouraged, but didn't push; some might say his nourishment created a monster!

Growing up, I was never what one would call a "jock." I have vague memories of my mother tuning in to Jack Lalanne's calisthenics on television; perhaps I absorbed subconsciously some of his gospel of physical fitness. Still active and doing pull-ups at eighty-five years of age, he may have birthed this culture of athletes; he was certainly the mind behind working out with weights and what we call "aerobics." But the mentality of the era made being a cheerleader for the boys' teams more prestigious than being the lead scorer on any of the girls' teams. I credit summer camp for providing a setting where my appreciation of being physically active developed. I learned to love playing soccer and paddling a canoe. At school, I liked recess, especially dodge ball, and field day was fun because I got a blue ribbon in the broad jump. Team sports were my interest through high school, the team effort being as important to me as my individual performance.

During college, however, I became a real couch potato. I fulfilled my one physical education requirement by walking across campus in my raincoat (girls were not allowed to wear pants of any kind) to the small swimming pool where I would prove that I could tread water; the second semester I learned how to grip and swing a golf club; I don't believe there is any physical education requirement now.

What small level of fitness I had then was totally lost in my twenty's. I tried all kinds of diets to maintain my weight: liquids, grapefruit, low calorie, low carbohydrate.... And then there came marriage and job responsibilities and, before long, three little boys to look after. Briefly I tried the Royal Canadian exercise program, but didn't stick with it for long. An extra fifteen pounds settled in on my body.

Psychologists agree that change usually begins with planning rather than action. Setting goals and having a partner are important in the beginning phases of most exercise programs. Eventually, I joined a health club.

There was a baby sitter on site, and I became acquaint-
ed with other women who were exercising. We found
creative ways to entertain children and get a workout,
like letting the kids play in the sandbox in the infield
while we ran around the track. Or I would go for a run
while Johnny got ready for work and watched the kids.

Gradually I learned to say "no" to some of the
requests to serve on committees, and found faster and
easier ways of accomplishing projects to make time for
myself. Women especially have to distinguish between
priorities and excuses. (There will always be dishes to
wash!) We internalize a lot of guilt when we do things
for ourselves. I found that when I exercised I was at
peace and more efficient in all areas of my life, and I
learned that taking care of others didn't necessitate
neglecting myself!

Running, biking, and swimming appealed to me
because I really like to cook and to eat, and the idea of
burning so many calories (roughly 600 per hour) was
amazing. I started to enter local races with Johnny.
Small successes fueled my early enthusiasm, but my
competition was limited because not many women my
age were in the races. Even now, twenty years later, my
dad can quickly put me in my place by asking, "And how
many were in your age group?"

The triathlon event was started in California and
moved on to Hawaii, where the first official Ironman
race took place in 1978 with twelve men participating;
the theory behind the competition was to settle finally
the ongoing argument between swimmers, cyclists, and
runners over who was the fittest. The first woman
crossed the finish line the next year. Our triathlon in
Nashville, the Music City Triathlon, which dates back
to 1979, has the distinction of being the second oldest

official multi-sport race in the U.S., perhaps in the world. Tremendous interest in the sport was generated by ABC's Wide World of Sports in 1982 when Julie Moss crawled across the finish line in Hawaii for all the world to see. During the 1980's and 1990's the sport grew phenomenally, and race budgets run well into seven figures. Thousands of triathlons are now staged around the world, often unique in distances and courses. However, certain things are universal in all races: once the initial gun sounds, the clock ticks continually. Fast transitions from the swim to the bike and the bike to the run are as crucial as being fast in each sport. Strategy is a factor, as are hydration and equipment. A rack of bikes at the race in Perth would purchase a plush automobile.

Much of the fun of my involvement stems from the friendships I've made with women of all ages. Locally, I have a group with whom I train and compete. We push each other to grow stronger and encourage each person's triumphs. We share training and racing secrets, as well as relax together. On a hot summer day, we'll think nothing of riding 40 to 70 miles on the bike, then stopping for a country breakfast of pancakes and eggs. Most residents of Nashville have never been to Santa Fe, Fly, or Boston (little communities out of the city). One friend, Liz, has been known to tell her office that she "had business in Boston" and would be in late to work that day. Of course, we're strongly competitive on race day.

This camaraderie extends to women from other cities whom I meet at races. At big competitions such as the World Championships, there are breakfasts hosted for women competitors. Dottie was one of the speakers at the breakfast in Perth; we had met at "World's" in Gold Coast, Australia, in 1991. She's in her seventies (still competing and looking great!) and has started a mentoring program to support and encourage women getting started in the sport. She reported to the audience that shoes, bicycles, helmets and clothing had been sent to third world countries where young girls would be equipped.

For myself and many fellow athletes, the relationship of mentoring is loose and can have many parameters, from taking a bike ride together to offering simple advice. I hope to give back in such ways, for I have gained tremendous life lessons, as well as a very strong and healthy body, from my involvement in these sports. By telling this story I hope to encourage others to become involved.

>—‹+›—O—‹+›—‹

Race day in Perth slowly approached. I was not training as much as I had been; "tapering" is the rule during the last five to six days before a race, but I was tapering a little more than I had planned. One day I swam a little at one of the fabulous facilities so common in that country which celebrates amphibianism (over 90% of Aussies live within ten miles of the sea). The complex had two 50-meter pools and two 25-meter pools, one of each outside, as well as weight machines, hot tubs, slides for the kids, and a shop with more brands of goggles and workout clothes than I had ever seen. One day I jogged and chatted with a group for forty-five minutes on the bike/running path which went for miles and miles all around the city and along the river. The women in my age group met at 6:45 the next morning and swam in the river to mimic race morning. I was in the water for only twelve to fifteen minutes, but there were a lot of people practicing, and I gained confidence that I could survive the swim.

Seeing the facilities in Australia and learning their attitudes toward exercise and fitness were inspiring. The Aussies were dominating many sports, including the triathlon, and it was obvious why. Our country has much to learn about encouraging our increasingly overweight population to get in shape; many states no longer require our children to take physical education. The percentage of obese children has grown from single to double digits in the last thirty years. We need to focus our efforts on the youngest members of society, creating an environment which enhances children's enjoyment of movement and their perception of physical competence. Active children become active adults; one can refer to www.pe4life.org for suggestions on advocacy for more and better physical education in the schools. Recent studies suggest that as many as 55% of Americans are now overweight or obese.

To determine a person's desirable weight, the American Heart Association uses the body mass index (BMI), which is calculated as weight in kilograms (weight in pounds divided by 2.2), divided by height in meters (height in inches multiplied by 0.0254) squared. (Don't groan: grab a pencil with a good eraser and exercise your brain with some long division and recall how to count decimal places! Hint: do a little "rounding off" ... remember how?) For example, I weigh roughly 118 pounds (53.6 kilograms), and I am 5 feet 3 1/2 inches tall (1.61 meters). First multiply 1.61 by itself; the result is 2.59. Then divide 53.6 by 2.59; the result of 20.69 can be rounded up to a BMI of 21. A BMI falling between 19 and 25 means that weight-related health risks are negligible, and one between twenty-five and thirty is considered overweight. A BMI of thirty or above indicates obesity. (See Appendix 2). Another gage of being too heavy is the waist-to-hip ratio (WHR). Simply divide the circumference of the waist by that of the hips. A result of less than 0.80 is desirable.

There is convincing proof that obesity contributes to many health problems, from diabetes to cardiovascular and joint disease. Studies also suggest that overweight women suffer from poor self image and even have suicidal thoughts more frequently than women of normal weight. It is important to remember, however, that BMI guidelines are just guidelines, and many women who work out consistently for years may never resemble those sleek elite athletes at world-championship events. The formula does not take into account an individual's heredity or body composition, a measure of muscle versus fat. A more accurate analysis may be determined with underwater weighing or tests using infrared equipment and electrical impedance. Regardless, expectations should be realistic and goals appropriate.

New studies hint that in terms of mortality, being "fit" may actually be more important than being "thin." A BMI less than nineteen is considered in the "danger zone" of malnutrition! And just as obesity is a public health threat, so are the consequences of eating disorders, especially among girls and women in America who are barraged with a daily dose of underweight models and actresses - all visions of perfection. Anorexia nervosa, defined as a weight less than 85% of what is considered normal for one's age and height, can lead to damage of the heart and kidneys and even death. Bulimia nervosa is more common than anorexia, occurring in two to four percent of all girls and women; this statistic is most likely very seriously under-reported. The pattern in bulimia is one of binging and purging, either by vomiting or use of laxatives. Long-term consequences can include damage to vital organs, as well as to tooth enamel, and, like any situation where one senses a personal loss of control, diminished self esteem.

The idea that there are now Web sites promoting starvation and glamorizing the illnesses is appalling. The main culprit leading to these disorders is dieting! I know how insidious the pattern can be, because I dealt with these issues for a time as a young woman. I counted every calorie and weighed my food; I wondered why I experienced irregular periods and subsequent infertility. One day I woke up and realized how foolish my behavior was. Exercise provided a healthy alternative to my perceived weight problems and a lifelong solution.

Many women become consumed by the weight loss and gain cycle of frequent dieting; we are duped by claims that certain food substitutes or supplements will make us lose several dress sizes in just two weeks! Whether it's ultra-metabolean, mega-lipofirm, or just "plain, pure water," frequent dieting of any kind makes it harder to lose weight and easier to gain, because our metabolism actually slows down and goes into starvation mode, in an effort to conserve energy. A healthy diet, in which no calories are counted nor food weighed, coupled with a lifestyle including plenty of physical activity can take us out of the pharmacies and doctors' offices.

Being moderately active on most, or even better on all, days of the week (i.e., thirty minutes of accumulated activity in a day) is especially important for the baby boomers. Failure to watch our diet and to pursue a regular exercise program will result in an increase in body fat and weight every year as we age. Not only will exercise prevent many disease processes, but it can also give us the ability to maintain an independent lifestyle and increases the likelihood that we'll enjoy our post-retirement years. There are virtually no contraindications to exercise. If weight loss is needed, it may take an hour a day of exercise to shed unwanted pounds. But don't let a perceived lack of skills be a stumbling block - all you need is to be able to move around! (see Appendix 1)

>-ı-+)-•-O-•-(+-ı-<

Two days before race day I attended the mandatory team meeting, led by the team manager Tim. This sent me, usually pretty calm, into a state of hot flashes and wet palms even though I had done my "homework" - that is, my training.

Because I have been doing this sport for many years, it has become a lifestyle. For years I kept a diary of my workouts, but I find this no longer necessary; either I'm less compulsive, or I know intuitively what I need to do. It is a rare day when I do not engage in some form of exercise. I swim, bike, or run, or a combination of these, every day; some days it may amount to only a four mile run, but most days I spend more than an hour or two at "working out." Weekend days usually involve long bike rides or runs. I run in just about any kind of weather (layering, tights, hats, gloves, and a good Goretex suit are invaluable). A gentle drizzle which lured me out to run sometimes becomes a torrential downpour. But a hot shower, making my skin red and prickly and a bowl of hot soup which warms the part of me unreached by the shower, can make a day special. I come inside to bike on a stationary bicycle, rather than riding outside, if the temperature is below fifty degrees or if it is raining.

Since I had qualified for the race in Perth, I had made only one change in my training. I had never before had a "personal trainer," but I had decided that an educated approach to total strength might provide an edge. Once a month I met with Matt who was recommended by my master's swim coach Carol, a past Olympian from

Canada. He gave me a set of exercises to enhance "core" body strength, as well as upper and lower body exercises with weights.

There are many myths surrounding strength training, especially among women. Many women are intimidated or think that they will become too muscular; this is simply not true! The weight room of the health club or the local YMCA is not the strict domain of body-builders. Working out with weights actually offers the best chance for redefining how your body looks at ANY age. It burns calories and improves bone density. I hoped that strength, or resistance, training would develop my muscles to generate more power and make me less prone to ligament and tendon injuries; thus I had added these exercises to my usual routine about twice a week.

Manager Tim wanted to be sure that we followed all the rules to avoid penalties and possible disqualification. I listened carefully. It was likely that wetsuits would be allowed because of the water temperature (relief). A review of the map clarified the three bike loops, pointing out the speed bumps on the road ("it might not be a good idea to 'bunny-hop' these if you don't want to 'flat'"), but even Tim was confused about the two and a half run loops. Promises were made to post a note on the board in the hotel lobby once he got clarification on the run course. We had to take our bikes to the race site the day before the race, where they would be checked for any unsafe equipment and left overnight.

An announcement was made that there would be random drug testing. I was not familiar with the whole long list of what they look for, but this was one further concern, leading to a discussion among some of the women in my age group, especially when they heard that I am a women's health nurse practitioner. One woman said emphatically, "I have decided not to take hormones. I'll go through 'the change' naturally" - to which I sheepishly ventured into a discussion of the benefits of hormone replacement therapy (HRT) - or, simply hormone therapy - and what she meant by "natural." Before the conversation was over, she wanted my e-mail address to continue our discourse.

Would my hormones result in a positive test if I were picked for a random drug test? After all the reading and studying I had done, I believed at that time that the benefits of HRT outweigh the risks. It had been shown in study after study that HRT definitely reduces loss of bone density (and therefore probably osteoporosis), probably heart disease (in women without preexisting disease), and perhaps many cancers as well. It provides better skin and urogenital tone and is hypothesized to reduce the occurrence of Alzheimer's and macular degeneration. The increased risk of breast cancer is slight, and those cancers appear to respond to treatment better among women who have a history of HRT use. What most women forget is that breast cancer is not the main killer of women, anyway - heart disease is. So I was taking a combination of estrogen, progesterone, and testosterone. The testosterone, a hormone produced by women's bodies as well as men's, falls off after menopause, just as do estrogen and progesterone. It appears that a little testosterone may boost a woman's bone strength, as well as her libido - that is, her interest in sex - and a feeling of well-being. It would require considerably more than I take to result in a deepening of the voice, facial hair, or other male characteristics.) At any rate, I decided that maybe I would leave off the testosterone before this race.... (See Appendix 5)

To prepare for the possibility of a hot day, I needed to start drinking extra water, to fill every cell maximally, but that meant more frequent trips to the "loo." "Carbo-loading," eating a larger percentage of carbohydrates in relationship to fats and protein to provide extra energy stores, was a hot topic among competitors. Much of the energy that an athlete uses comes from the breaking down of a substance called glycogen. It is made up of long pieces of glucose (carbohydrates) and is stored in our muscle and liver. There's only so much that our body can store. After about an hour and a half of hard physical effort, the glycogen is used up. The story of "hitting the wall" is not a fairy tale. At that point, the body shifts to body fat as its source of fuel. Fat is used more slowly as a fuel and causes the athlete to slow down. By eating extra carbs during the three days prior to the event, one can store glycogen at a higher level. Sports drinks, such as Gatorade, and energy bars during the event are very important in delaying fatigue. I believe the most reasonable piece of advice is not to overeat and not to eat unfamiliar things during the days preceding the race ... like kangaroo and pomegranates.

The day before a race always finds me fairly lethargic; my body is resting. It was no different in Perth. I jogged the few blocks down to the race site to look over the transition area and commit to memory where my small space would be. Crucial time could be lost if I didn't learn how many bike racks I would pass on the way in from the swim and the bike segments of the race. In smaller races, competitors put up balloons on their rack or use colored chalk on the pavement. This practice is not allowed at world events, so I counted and counted again the number of racks. Back in the hotel, I left messages with Karen, another woman on the team; she had a bike pump and I needed to get maximum pressure in my tires before taking the bike down. She didn't respond, so I asked someone else in our hotel lobby to borrow a pump. This accomplished, the bike was walked down and deposited in my spot, after passing inspection, with plastic bags tied over the seat and the computer in case of rain overnight. I had a "conversation" with my bike, filled with positive reinforcement, before leaving it. Security was very tight. All competitors had a race band on their wrists after registration (I felt like a hospital patient), and only competitors were allowed into the transition area.

I don't often take naps, but that afternoon was different - I slept like a puppy for over an hour. Good thing, because sleep the night before a race is usually fitful. Dinner was light - risotto with chicken, almonds, and pumpkin and one beer, plus water. We were in bed with lights out before 9 pm; the alarm was set for four in the morning. Several nocturnal trips to the bathroom were necessary with all the water I'd drunk.

Race morning dawned with a cool ocean breeze blowing through the open glass doors and birds singing. We were up and drinking coffee early. Johnny was on the medical team and he needed to tape one woman's wrist. She had had a bike wreck a month before and experienced pain while shifting gears.

A race is a mental and spiritual test, as well as a physical one. I said my favorite prayer - the Serenity Prayer of AA (Alcoholics Anonymous) - as far as I'm concerned a prayer for any occasion: "God grant me the serenity to accept those things I cannot change, the courage to change those things I can, and the wisdom to know the difference."

I consumed my usual pre-race breakfast about three hours before the start of the event: a large cup of cafe au lait (lowfat milk for protein), a banana, and a power bar, washed down with water and Gatorade. I walked down to the transition area in the dark with my bag of gear and began the process of setting up my essentials, making periodic trips to the portajohn. My age category was written in waterproof ink on my right calf; I was an "H" which indicated women 50 to 54. My timing "chip," the size of a quarter, was on a strap secured with Velcro around my right ankle; every time I passed over a timing mat, a computer record would be made. After putting the strap on too tightly at one race, resulting in a bloody ankle, I took care. Pictures were flashed and last minute mental notes registered, when suddenly it was time to head for the start of the swim.

I was in the third "wave" with about 120 women over 45, starting five minutes after the second wave. We slid into the water off a pier on cue and quickly became a great female "mosh pit" of green swim caps, black wetsuits and flailing arms. I tried to stay on the fringe of the group to avoid the likelihood that a faster swimmer would come groping over me. This was comfortable, but about ten minutes into the event I felt something large, fleshy and weird with my right hand as I stroked under my pelvis; quick assessment had me debating whether it was a drowned swimmer from a previous wave or a shark. I gasped and quickly sprinted in closer to the main group. (I'll never outswim a shark, but like two hikers running from a bear, it's best to beat the other hiker!) There were no unaccounted-for swimmers after the race and no sharks sighted in the river, which is several miles in from the sea; surely then what I felt was a large jellyfish.

A large sun rose over the city at dawn in a burning-red welcome as I rounded the final buoy heading for the shore. I pulled off my goggles and cap as I ran up and over the steep ramp into the transition area. I reached my bike with the back zipper already pulled down on the wetsuit, but getting the suit off over my ankles was like dealing with glue. I tugged as folds stuck to folds and caught on the timing device around my ankle. Quick words of exasperation were shared with other competitors also having this problem. Precious time was lost, adrenalin was wasted, and this realization registered in my mind: hours upon hours had been devoted to swimming, biking, and running; why hadn't I practiced taking off my wetsuit?

After what seemed an eternity, the first loop on the bike finally began. My bike was performing beautifully; she and I climbed the infamous Malcolm hill and sped through the park as my breathing became even, and I sipped some fluid. I passed an Aussie with an "H" and caught Ramona as we finished the first loop, making no eye contact. One Aussie "H" zipped past me at breakneck speed, and I thought I might have seen Rita go by on her red bike. I was pretty confident that none of the other nine Americans in my age group were ahead of us, but I had no idea about those from other countries; I hadn't noticed how many bikes close to mine were already out of transition, and I hadn't met any of these other women (second mistake of the day). I was not willing to test my aerobic threshold by passing Ramona and decided to ride even with her. She and I rode neck and neck the rest of the way. Riding hard, I dedicated each lap to someone who had helped me train smarter during the last six months. Shockingly, the last corner was upon us, and we skidded to the grassy finish, leaving rubber on the pavement like a controlled slide in a NASCAR race.

This transition was much faster than my first, thank goodness; the racing flats were on my feet, and my spirit as a runner was tapped. Out on the course I felt good, keeping Ramona about fifteen yards ahead. I knew that going out too fast would be a mistake, so I hung back, maintaining the distance. I saw all of the other Americans in the "H" group behind me as I rounded the turn of the first loop (I know them all - and we were all wearing the USA team swimsuit). Rita was there, too, so it hadn't been her red bike after all. Ramona and I maintained the same pace, grabbing water at each aid station for a gulp and short splash before throwing the cup to the side, not slowing down at all. Mile markers were not given, of course, because this race was in kilometers, so I did not know my per-mile pace. My past experience with perceived effort told me enough, though, and I could not catch Ramona. We both went by an Aussie "H" with the finish line in sight, so I experienced another "red line" finish. I hung my head briefly to catch my breath and walk a few steps, embraced Ramona with a mutually-friendly, endorphin-filled "good race" hug and moved immediately into comparative stories about the race. I had finished in two hours 36 minutes, with her about twenty seconds ahead.

Neither of us knew then that there were in fact nine women in our age group ahead of her, six of us within a span of two minutes. Oh, sharp regrets over not practicing the wetsuit removal! And regrets of not taking the risk to pass Ramona during the bike ride haunted me, too. Yes, hindsight is always perfect vision.

I had seen my weaknesses and would work on correcting them. Champions have an uncanny confidence and optimism and know that most races are half physical and half mental. A positive self-image, as well as determination and mental toughness, can turn an athletic challenge into a powerful performance. I was in fact pleased to have improved my time by ten minutes from the qualifying race six months before, on a very similar course, and to have been the second American in my age group. I know that each finish line is temporary; each end not a real end. This is just life, and its players go on to yet another starting horn and another transition, another hard effort and feeling of satisfaction, if not a perfect race. In a year and a half I would "age up" to the 55-59 group. I would have won that age group with my time in the race in Perth!

The awards dinner was upbeat, replete with good food, address swaps and promises to keep in touch. An Aussie approached me with her friend and asked, "We are close to the same size, would you exchange jackets with me?" I had many other pieces from the USA uniform as mementos, so we autographed one another's jackets, inside on the lining, and said goodbye, wearing our opponent's clothes!

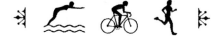

May 2000

*"Travel is fatal to prejudice, bigotry,
and narrow-mindedness."*

Mark Twain

"We will make this an extended trip. I will take off four weeks, and we'll make it kind of a sabbatical, in celebration of my not taking any more 'night call'." This was Johnny's reaction as soon as I had qualified to be on the American team for the World Championships in Australia. (At the age of 55, all members of his orthopaedic group give up their responsibility of taking emergency call on weekends and nights, so he would not have to ask anyone to cover for him.) In 1991, we had made the trip to Gold Coast, north of Sydney, and stayed only ten days, barely long enough to do the race and recover from jet lag before returning home - not adequate time to take advantage of such a long journey!

I understood his feelings; he had been working long hours in the demanding profession of surgery for over 25 years. Only twice before had we been gone for more than two weeks at a time. With the three boys away, this was a perfect time. Of course the biggest problem was that while away from his practice, Johnny would not be drawing any income - doctors are providers of services - no work, no pay. I enjoyed my job as a nurse practitioner, and although part time, it did contribute financially and would also probably be jeopardized by such an extended "holiday." There was the added concern of being so far away from elderly parents and even older

41

children; in short, the decision was not simple. We spent weeks weighing the pros and cons.

At the same time, several of our training buddies were discussing a triathlon which they were planning to do in Kona, Hawaii, four weeks after my race in Perth. "Come on, Emily, you might as well stop over in Hawaii and do this race (as if Hawaii was just around the block)." I was tempted. During the last year I had done three triathlons which were qualifiers for the famous Hawaiian Ironman. In my age group, you must finish first to qualify, and I had missed qualifying by only one place three times! I had done the Ironman in 1987 and had not really tried to qualify again until last year, as my post-race feelings in 1987 were similar to a mother's reaction right after delivering a baby - "I don't want to do that ever again, at least not any time soon." But those feelings had somehow faded, as they obviously do in the case of having babies. I was aware that through the years it has gotten more difficult to qualify, as more women have become involved as well as fit, and secondly there are fewer qualifying races. This particular race would be one of only four qualifying half-ironman distance races this year (all the rest are full distance - 2.4 mile swim, 112 mile bike ride and 26.2 mile run). I didn't care to do an ironman-distance race other than the one in Kona, now accepted as the World Championship Ironman! So, I was very tempted by my friends' suggestion.... The idea of being gone for five weeks seemed somehow irresponsible and frivolous, but I began to toy with it. The elusive return to the Hawaiian Ironman in October, 2000, had become a forbidden fruit, just beyond my reach. But how would I continue to train, and also enjoy the trip, while traveling around after Perth? The time away would most likely signal a change in my career path, if not in Johnny's.

I had worked for six months to maximize my conditioning and had remained uninjured; I came to believe that not to do this would be to cheat myself. So, after a few phone calls to the travel agent with whom I was working, the decision was made to "go for it" - and buy adequate trip insurance! We planned the "trip of a lifetime," and then everyone who had expressed an interest in going along as cheerleaders in Perth and fellow trekkers backed out! It would be just the two of us.

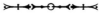

The morning following the race in Perth, we packed up the bicycle and left the modern city, flying into the "outback" region of Ayers Rock. The large crimson rock, known as Ularu by the natives, sits in a vast land of myths and legends and is a manifestation of this country's cultural diversity. As our group hiked around the base of the rock (it is considered sacrilegious to climb the rock, though many people do), local whites came along to interpret for the Aboriginal guides, who were friendly and proud but retiring. We soaked up the murky history of these people who have inhabited this land for at least 40,000 years, in comparison to the whites' 200. Quite poor by our standards and still lacking political clout, many Aborigines continue to live a seminomadic existence in tribes and speak languages which are unintelligible to one another. But a traditional oral culture, based on their concept of a period called the Dreamtime, a circle of life into and from the earth, circling around and over the monolith itself, has remained amazingly consistent and continuous for centuries, passed down in pictures, dances, and songs. There are many social issues yet to be resolved by the blacks and whites Downunder.

Another glimpse into the land's many traditions was delivered by a cowboy poet from the back of a camel. He recited rhythmic words as he rode side-saddle, and the beast swayed below in a lumbering walk, periodically halting to snatch a bite of a green plant. Seeing the desert at sunset while straddling a camel was quite a different concept of exercise!

During the week in Perth, Johnny had noticed that a previously benign sebaceous cyst on his back had become inflamed; he thought he might have scraped it on some coral while snorkeling. In spite of taking anti-inflammatories and antibiotics for four days, the lump looked angrier than ever. We felt that it needed to be lanced and drained; I wondered if we might have to go home. He wanted me to drain it, but I did not have the experience or the appropriate instruments, so we searched out the emergency health care clinic in the tiny desert town, where a nurse practitioner did an amazingly competent job.

"Hold on to the table," he warned, right before he lanced deeply into my husband's back with his scalpel. With no anesthesia, he offered only moral support. After the surgery, we were given a tour of the facility and learned how the Royal Flying Medical Doctors attempt to provide coverage to this large diverse continent. The practitioner told us of his delivery of twins the week before to a 13-year old Aboriginal girl. We paid our $50 bill (seemed a bargain to me!) and returned a few hours later with gifts for the kind, efficient staff. I irrigated the wound and changed his dressings daily, the wound healing nicely as we continued our travels.

On to New Zealand, where we toured the south island, dodging sheep as they moved from one grassy field to graze another and feeling the spray of waterfalls spilling over narrow, winding roads. My scant training consisted of a few runs and thirty minutes on a wobbly stationery bike.

Trainer Matt had put together a series of resistance exercises for me to do with long rubber bands made for this purpose, as well as stretching and core strength-type exercises, such as pushups. I knew that, if I wanted to stay active, stretching and flexibility exercises should demand more of my attention as I aged - yoga or Pilates would be a good addition to my present program. Older bodies become less flexible and are more prone to injury; well-stretched muscles reduce post-exercise aches and pains, help manage stress, and improve our posture and our circulation. Matt's workouts were easy compared to what I had been doing at home.

Detailed itineraries had been prepared and sent to family members before the trip, and I had made arrangements for a reasonably priced international phone calling card, but we had been staying in touch mostly by e-mail. Connections were easy in Perth, but during the three days we were in the "outback," we were never able to get online. Once I logged on in Christchurch, New Zealand, I found a very upsetting message from Keith, our 20-year old son. "Will is doing OK after his surgery ... he's a tough kid." My heart sank; this had to be a joke. Scanning back, there was a two-day-old message from Keith saying that Will, our 18-year old son who is a competitive snowboarder, had "broken his leg." Only two months before, we had watched, with our hearts in our throats, as he had beautifully executed frontside corkscrews, rodeos, and 720's as ESPN filmed in Lake Tahoe. His pride at placing fourth in a national competition and receiving his first large cash purse was thrilling for all of us.

We knew Will was to be in California for a photo shoot. Since he was 18, parental permission for surgery was unnecessary, and he had screws put in for a tibial plateau fracture right after the accident. After many frantic phone calls, we finally got in touch with the surgeon, whose report was extremely disturbing to Johnny. The doctor, who drives four hours up from LA to cover mountain accidents on weekends, couldn't remember the details of Will's case and wouldn't have access to his records until he went back in two days. He had treated another snowboard injury the same day and had the injuries confused; the one he recalled sounded horrible.

Johnny confided, "It sounds like one of the worst automobile accidents I've ever seen in my practice; he'll definitely have arthritis from this." Up until that moment of discovery on my laptop, I had been free as a bird - laughing, running, smiling, floating in the south Pacific. I began to wonder whether I needed to go be with Will; the previous fall I had gone to help Keith when he had an emergency appendectomy. Maybe we needed to activate the trip insurance. It's terrible being so far away when your child is hurt; I cried.

We finally located Will and were somewhat relieved just to hear his voice; his two friends, Charlie and Scott, were taking care of him. When we had our follow-up call with the surgeon, records now in hand, he apologized that he had been thinking of the other boy's accident; Will's was not quite as bad. Will knew the other boy; he'd done a 50-foot jump and landed on the flats. Will was doing tricks on "a rail" in the snowpark, and the rail fell over, twisting his board and yanking his leg ("I promise I didn't do anything stupid, Mom"). The officials at the mountain resort had removed the rails the next day. We discussed the importance of his following the doctor's instructions and rehab to the letter; during the next days we talked frequently, but I didn't go home. In my haste, I had failed to send an itinerary to Keith; in his haste, Will had not taken his itinerary to California with him. Of course if this had been a life and death matter, they assured me, they would have found us by phone.

>–⊷–◦–⊶–◅

We continued our sojourn. Our next stop was tropical Fiji; we were so different from the worldly, jet-setting baby-boomers who might be visiting this exotic place! We looked more like the "Snopes" family in Faulkner, carting all our gear around with us, lugging the bike box, packed with a bike pump, shoes, helmet, and plastic bags of dirty clothes, backpacks slung over our shoulders. When the bike box was declared over the weight limit, we squatted on the floor of the airport in New Zealand rearranging the contents of our luggage for all to see. We breathed a false sigh of relief after we made some adjustments in our packing.

"Lady, let me see your carry-on," muttered the security guard, demanding much respect with his pistol and his I-mean-business stance, as we had our bags scanned before heading to our gate. "You cannot carry these aboard the aircraft." He was holding up the two small CO_2 cartridges which I had finally found in Australia, in short supply because of the plethora of athletes at the world championship. The cartridges provide a quick way of inflating a tire after changing a flat. I wanted to save them for Hawaii and felt it was safer not to pack them in our checked luggage. He confiscated the cartridges, and we were required to fill out a form admitting that we had attempted to take a dangerous object aboard an aircraft; however, we were then allowed to go to our flight. I felt as if I had been reprimanded by a stern school teacher!

We enjoy scuba diving and are certified, so we had booked five nights on an island with wonderful access to diving. Breathing compressed air as slowly as possible to conserve oxygen while leisurely watching lovely fish definitely stretches the definition of "cross training"! The concept of "cross training" is relatively new. By alternating athletic activities, the theory goes, opposing muscles are stressed, lessening the likelihood of injury. Most serious athletes in any sport these days do some form of cross-training. But in triathlon, it's really rather redundant to speak of cross training, for our sport is defined as multi-sport.

In addition to our four morning dives, we paddled a sea kayak the three miles around the island one afternoon and swam around it with flippers the other afternoon. Necessity being "the mother of invention," I also ran repeats of the steps from the beach up to the ridge where our thatched hut was located. The native Fijians, gentle, soft-spoken, and slow-moving, thought I was a bit crazed; I definitely made an impression. As it happened, the best training I had in Fiji had nothing to do with workouts. Heat adaptation takes two to three weeks; the race in Hawaii would be run in extremely hot weather, so the tropical temperature in an unairconditioned hut in Fiji was what I needed! We spent our final morning touring a native Fijian village and talking to one of their chiefs. We conversed at length about the amicable relationship between the natives and the Indian residents who came to help with the sugar cane industry in the late 1800s.

>━┤◆>━○━<◆┤━<

Finally we headed to Hawaii, and, back in the USA, I felt close to home, in spite of the pounding surf off my balcony. Two days after our arrival, we heard that there had been a political coup in Fiji, and that Americans were advised not to travel there! We were shocked and horrified.

Kona, on the Big Island, had been a sleepy town with a single traffic light when we had been there in 1987. Because of the international publicity associated with the Ironman, the city is now besieged with athletes who live and train there year-round, as well as lots of tourists and a large contingent of retirees. It was still fun to be back and stay in the same little "hole-in-the-wall" hotel where we had stayed in 1987. We remembered so well the tide pool right next to us, where our boys, then aged five, seven, and ten, learned to snorkel. The bakery where I had indulged in my huge "Ironman" donuts was gone.

Memories of that 1987 trip filled my mind and heart.... I had come to the Big Island a week early, before my family, to recover from jet lag, learn the course of the Ironman race, and to train. I had entered that race with only one goal - to finish. I had done each separate event individually; that is, I had swum 2.4 miles, biked 112 miles, and run numerous marathons. But I had never done them all in the same day! This is a grueling combination, to be sure. We had watched the race two years before when Johnny was there for a medical meeting. We were both doing shorter races at that time, but this was a different beast. We looked at each other as we stood sweating and cheering for the athletes running in the searing afternoon sun and said, simultaneously, "I'll never do this race!" The following year I qualified for an

Ironman slot at the "Crawfishman" triathlon in Louisiana and prepared to "eat my words." The day of that Ironman race in October of 1987, will always be a high point in my life, rating in excitement with the three days my sons came into this world.

I'll never forget several very special moments during that week in 1987. The masters (over age 40) women's breakfast was held in a home up in the hills overlooking the town of Kona. We sat at picnic tables under the banyan trees, as several veterans gave the newcomers their pearls of advice. The scene was tasteful and feminine, but the tip I had been waiting for (but was afraid to ask) came: "You need to know how to pee on the bike...." Many of us first-timers were perplexed, because you never get off your bike during a race unless you must change a flat tire. There are no portajohns out on the course or even bushes behind which to squat, and, besides, the clock is ticking! This veteran described it clearly for us: "Raise up off your seat with your feet parallel, grip the top tube with your quads, concentrate, and let 'er rip! At the next aid station, take a water bottle and splash yourself." I broke the "don't ever try anything new on race day" rule with that one - a necessity!

There were get-togethers during the week leading up to the big event for swims from the pier where the race starts in town, pancake breakfasts, and other social gatherings. I trained, and I ate. I discovered the shop that sold "Ironman" donuts and indulged in the monstrous sweet creations, laden with carbohydrates (and plenty of fat!) I bet I gained seven to eight pounds that week, as I tapered my workouts the last five days (certainly the only time I have ever tried to gain weight!). My husband and three boys arrived two days before the event, with a beautiful red rose from my rose garden. I was ready.

Race day on that October morning in 1987 dawned sunny. We were body-marked (I was #250), and 1,200 swimmers started *en masse* at seven in the morning, as helicopters flew overhead filming for television. I remember looking through my goggles to see the colorful fish swimming below and seeing scuba divers with cameras on the ocean floor as well. My race went as planned; I stayed in control of my fluids and ate the fig newtons stashed in my shirt pocket while I biked (energy bars weren't around then). The winds were as vicious as I had heard - the rumor was that people have been blown off their bikes. So the advice was this: "Grip your top tube with your quads as you come down from Hawi (the turn-around of the bike ride). It'll make you feel one with your bike." When I finished the bike ride and started to run, the sun was low in the sky, so I was blessed with shade. It had been so hot on the bike out on the Queen Kamehameha Highway, with the asphalt of the highway and black lava fields as a landscape in all directions, absorbing all that heat. People later said there had been spectators frying eggs on the pavement!

My run went well. I walked through the aid stations, where I got cold sponges, water, and de-fizzed coke, which provides caffeine for a quick lift. I remember one particular aid station after it got dark that day. I thought that I was at mile twenty-one; when I asked the volunteer for validation, she said, "No, you are at mile seventeen." Downtrodden and sure I was right, I argued. Finally, I realized that they (the volunteers) should know, and I went on. The finish line was glorious. Johnny and the boys were there, and to this day I regret that I didn't encourage the boys to cross the finish line with me, which would have been permitted. After all, they had been my spirit and my encouragement. But something within me made me finish this thing the way

I had started it - alone. It had been a very long day of racing: twelve hours and nineteen minutes.

When I finished and received my lei, I thought that I felt fine, but after a few minutes, I slumped to the ground. A little massage and a hamburger (there's something about hot meat which always appeals to me after a hard effort) brought me around, and we walked the mile back to the hotel. Despite the overwhelming exhaustion, I could not sleep that night. My metabolism was wacky, and my senses were on fire, so I sat on the balcony for several hours thinking about my experience. The next day I collected my bike and learned that I had placed fifth in my age group and would earn a medal! The family had planned to take a boat trip to snorkel; I went, but was walking very slowly. While they snorkeled, I floated in a tube and sipped a Mai-Tai. My number had been written in indelible ink, and the rest of me was covered with sunscreen. For a month after the race, the "250" remained a tattoo on both my upper arms and my quads.

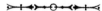

I had done little real training during the previous three weeks after leaving Perth and was nervous and anxious to get started, as I knew well that muscle strength and fitness level can be maintained about this long before an athlete begins to lose ground. Johnny rented a road bike from a local shop (we had not taken his bicycle because of the hassle of hauling bikes around on trains, cars, and planes). He did two rides, two swims, and one long run with me before he flew back home to get back to work. I had eleven days until the 2000 Keauhou-Kona Triathlon.

The ocean swims from the pier in town were delightful. There were no waves rolling in, although the surf could be choppy with swells, and the water was clear enough to see all kinds of colorful fish (as well as big turtles and coral the hues of the rainbow). There would be no wetsuits in this race, the water temperature being quite comfortable. The swimming area was parallel to the shore and was well marked by buoys and respected by boaters. Lots of locals swam there every morning, granting a degree of safety.

I have become more comfortable in the water, as well as faster and more efficient, since I started swimming regularly with a masters' swim class. These groups for all ages and levels of ability exist throughout the country and are definitely the best way to improve form and boost confidence. Though it is difficult to master superior technique when one is learning as an adult, swimming is a marvelous way to maintain flexibility and get an aerobic workout without the pounding generated by gravity while running and, to a lesser degree, by biking. The sport tones upper body muscles, minimizing a sagging chin and underarm flab, and provides wonderful flexibility for the neck. I recommend learning to breathe bilaterally, that is, on both sides, when doing the freestyle stroke, even though everyone prefers one side over the other. It must be said, however, that as a non-weight-bearing activity, swimming does nothing to maintain bone density, and thus needs to be only one part of a program which includes weight-bearing activities.

One morning down at the pier, I saw the trademark "design" on a man's left shoulder. He looked like a pretty conservative kind of guy; "I'm in investments in San Francisco and can't afford for my boss or my clients to see my tattoo when I'm dressed in a suit." The Ironman logo is an "m," super-imposed on an "i," with the dot above. Most people with this tattoo have done the Ironman, though of course anyone can get the tattoo, whether they've done the race or not. Last year Marti, who has also done the Ironman, came up to me at a race and said, "You, Kathleen, and I ought to get the Ironman tattoo." I had preached to my boys since they were little about not getting tattoos - "don't do anything permanent to your body that you might regret later in life". I had been disheartened when my eldest son John got one; but I had seen tattoos all the time in my practice. Ray, who has numerous tattoos, encouraged me, "Em, the world is different now." And Liz got one this year.... I was tempted; I could get one in a spot where no one (except my husband!) would know about it until I'm dead or beyond caring who knows .... The Big Island Tattoo Shop was only four blocks away ... surely they used sterile, safe practices. But I just kept thinking of one of my patients. The middle-aged woman is now a church secretary; she sorely regrets the roses, the "I'm yours," the hearts and arrows, and the Harley emblem which run up and down her arms and legs ....

The Queen Kamehameha Highway, where triathlons go out and back, ran sixty miles north along the coast from Kona to the end of the Big Island at Hawi. It was smooth and had a very wide shoulder for all the cyclists. There were no billboards and very little litter. The scenery was almost beyond description. The Big Island is a volcanic island, with Mauna Loa and Mauna Kea each over 13,000 feet. Kilauea, at the south end of the island, has been erupting since 1983 and was still spilling lava into the sea, but the devastation and scenery along this northern section dated back to an 1859 flow. The landscape was covered with lava, huge black chunks of rock, with older flow areas birthing a new life of tan and green-stalked wild grasses which blew in the constant ocean breezes; there were no trees, but occasional splashes of wild bougainvillea bushes of fluorescent red, pink, white and orange. To one side green hills rose to Mauna Kea, often shrouded in clouds and snow-covered in winter, and to the horizon on the other side was the blue ocean, mottled from light to dark.

Johnny's and my first ride was ten miles out and ten back, and there was very little wind, which is rare; we allowed ourselves to be fooled. The next day, we rode twenty-five miles out and turned to fight a fierce head-wind for the twenty-five mile ride back. One good rule for biking, and also for running, is to go out against the wind, so that the return will be blessed by a tailwind. Unfortunately, our route didn't work that way in Hawaii - the wind was out of the south 90% of the time!

I completed two more long rides by myself. The easy ride out allowed for a lot of daydreaming and contemplation of a new, but actually quite pleasing, form of graffiti along the lunar-like landscape. There were the usual messages such as "Jane loves David," "I love Tory," and "in loving memory of Rick," as well as "Happy Anniversary" and "Aloha," but they were written with bleached-white coral rocks laid on the lava. I found myself wondering if Jane and David were still together, and if Rick's ashes had been dropped at sea or if he was buried under the mound of lava along the road. Then there was a form of advertising - a large group of rocks spelled out "Toshiba," and one said "Asics." The latter one was gone on my last ride, but there was no "Nike" in its place. I mused that there had been "Mary loves Tom" and that maybe Jane and David came late one night and used the rocks to write their own names! I hoped no one would take up the "in loving memory of..." messages, though. I found myself mulling over a hidden meaning in some of them, like the letters on license plates. What did "swing plain" mean, and did "END" signal the end of a relationship or a suicide threat? Did the writer of "Got water?" die of thirst? The message written by "Genius," perfectly straight and large, was the easiest to read as I rode; I bet she or he had scored 1600 on the SATs!

There was a sign warning for donkeys crossing the road at dawn and at dusk. I would love to have seen them, but I never did. Turning back into the headwind made me stop my random musings and concentrate on the ride, get down and stay as aerodynamic as possible! During the last thirty minutes of a ride I'm usually planning what I will eat when I get back and what I will do for the rest of the day.

➤─┤◆➤─O─◄◆├─◄

I started serious bicycle riding when I became interested in triathlons and soon discovered exercise and touring to be a wonderful combination. Distance riding in southern France, Ireland, Colorado, and Vermont has provided a unique way to see different cultures - I hope to enjoy this for the rest of my life. My sister-in-law took one look at my racing bike and said, "That looks like the most uncomfortable thing imaginable." Actually, it is very comfortable. Two things make a bicycle comfortable: the right size bike "fit" by a bicycle shop, with the seat at the correct level to avoid knee problems, and a saddle made especially for women, with a hole in the middle! Before I got mine, I would grit my teeth in the shower from being rubbed raw between the legs.

While feeling the breeze blow through your hair is exhilarating, a helmet is essential. For anyone who continues to ride, it's not a matter of if you will have a wreck but when. Most riders I know have had at least one spill, some quite serious. I hit a dog one day when I misjudged his intentions, flipping over my handlebars and landing on my shoulder and head. I was "out" briefly, but my helmet, which cracked, probably prevented a more severe injury. Even Lance Armstrong, with multiple wins of the Tour de France, broke a vertebra in his neck after a downhill, blind-curve collision that destroyed his bike and helmet. Furthermore, wearing earphones is not a good idea; a cyclist needs all senses to ride defensively. Any level rider can get good advice from people at the bike shops, who also usually know about group rides.

>—¡‹›•‹›•O•‹›•¡‹

The run segment of the Kona triathlon went south through the village, and I staged my training runs along this route, right out the door of my hotel. The road courses along the shore, where surfers take advantage of big waves and snorkelers paddle face down in the sandy bays. Walls of neatly cut and stacked black lava rocks, draped with lovely hanging branches of flowering bougainvillea, border hotels, homes, and outdoor markets. Palm trees provide welcome shade, and the thick roots and huge size of stately banyan trees speak of longevity. Pairs of tiny yellow birds flicker, and the fragrance of frangipani occasionally floats by.

In spite of the ideal setting, I was having some troubles: the rubber nose bridge of my sunglasses was coming loose on one side when I started sweating, which happened quickly there. I needed a solution to that exasperating problem, as well as a remedy for a blister on one of my toes - things weren't perfect even in "Paradise"!

My increased exercise during the week had left me quite tired and my muscles tight, and I treated myself to a massage. I don't get massages regularly, partly because I don't want to take the time, but partly because I feel they are extravagant. However, when one is training intensely, the process does soothe overworked muscles and probably contributes to injury prevention. The incredible value of touch to human beings is widely recognized in today's stressful world, and it may be one of the oldest and simplest forms of medical treatment; it definitely makes me feel better. I presented myself to Leslie, therapist at the host hotel for the race, requesting a "sports massage."

My left shoulder hurt after I swam one day, so I didn't swim the following day; my left hip hurt after I ran that morning, so I wouldn't bike or run the next morning. Through the years I have experienced most of the "overuse injuries" - plantar fasciaitis, iliotibial-band syndrome, sore kneecaps, etc. Thus I have learned to "listen to my body." Truly, experience is the teacher whose lessons you remember the longest. I went for another massage and did some stretching!

Visiting the official web site of this event, I found the names and home cities of the other eleven women in my age group, as well as a list of those who had placed in the event for the last two years, with their times. I saw that #1 last year wasn't returning; #2 (Sally) would be there again. My anticipated times were very close to what she had done - but it was the others I knew nothing about who probably would be my main rivals.

When I called home, Keith sounded worried about his mother: "You mean you don't have any friends there?" I reassured him that I didn't know a soul in Kona but that I would be quite fine until the others arrived from Nashville. Actually, even though the locals had been friendly, I kept to my rituals for these prerace days and created a schedule to avoid loneliness. I spent time shopping, reading, writing, and sightseeing, as well as training. I followed winding, rocky paths leading to caves which had provided early nomadic people with shelter from the relentless trade winds and studied petroglyphs telling their stories. Visiting the Place of Refuge on the black lava flats of the southern Kona Coast was educational; I hoped it would imbue me with the legendary *mana* (spiritual power) of the Hawaiian royalty. I snapped pictures of the places. I took myself out for a date; we went to dinner and a movie. It seemed somewhat awkward to me, but it made me grateful for my family and friends at home. I got some Superglue for my sunglasses; the pain in my shoulder and hip and my blister were improving.

Three days til raceday. Ray and Gail arrived first. It was a good thing, because I had started talking to myself, and I was not sleeping very well. Ray warned, "All you can do by training during the last week is to hurt yourself." I believed him; he's finished Ironman five times! Ray and I swam briefly in the ocean and rode easily for about 45 minutes. Then the carbo-loading began - pancakes for brunch, pasta for dinner. The longer the race, the more important are the nutritional components before, during, and after the event. The goal is to take in 500 grams of carbohydrates during each of the three days prior to a race; complex carbohydrates like potatoes, rice, and bread are the best. One needs to drink until one "pees clear," and then keep drinking water, Gatorade, juice, whatever - but not much alcohol, which is dehydrating!

Then Rob, Melissa, Rusty, and Mary Ann arrived. Ray, Rob, and Rusty, "the 3 R's" - the guys who talked me into doing the race, were finally there! The excitement built. I showed them around since I had been there to check it all out. We ate more pancakes, omelettes, potatoes, bananas, fish, rice and ice cream; we kept drinking. We compared bike gearing, discussed how to defog goggles and whether to wear hats on the run, and so forth and so on. Many athletes were out training on the course, but we used the Br'er Rabbit technique (we "lay low"), and we kept eating and drinking. It was hot and sunny, and the ocean roared. Ray lost his goggles, and there was something wrong with Rob's bike when he put it together, so we made our third trip to the triathlon store in town.

It was Blast Off, minus one day. Taking care of last minute details, we went to register for the race, where we picked up our numbers and timing chips, and attended the mandatory pre-race meeting. Mary Ann bleached Rusty's hair; they made me agree to let them bleach mine if I won my age group. We were adults playing like kids, really. The sport attracts a highly motivated and driven subculture of men and women from all walks of life and careers. The ability to organize your time and balance your life are critical to the sport; there is also an undeniable desire to push the limits, to go a little harder, a little further, maybe to be a little "different...." Participants usually love the outdoor life; they aren't in it for the fame, definitely never for the money. Certainly, moments of creativity occur while working out, and the opportunity to "play" undeniably provides an escape from life's demands and obligations. But when one's heart is pounding and the primitive needs of air, water, and nourishment are paramount, other demands and obligations are moved to the back burner.

We continued to eat, drink, and tried to stay off our feet; the mood became increasingly solemn as we each began to focus on the difficult test of endurance, strength, training, strategy, and resolve facing us the following day. We chose carbohydrates that were more refined and were easier to digest; this was not the time for increasing fiber!

Race day. I was awakened by a nightmare at 3:45 a.m., something about a race - my alarm was set for 4 - and looked out to see stars. Starlit dawns are usually cause for delight, but not that day; we had been praying for clouds. My traditional breakfast was consumed, the call to the bathroom answered, and the Serenity Prayer whispered before the group assembled prior to daylight to drive to the race site. Gail, Mary Ann, and Melissa would drop us off, park, and return to help us lather up with sunscreen and take pictures. All the twenty-odd women over age fifty vying for the one Ironman slot (and out there to have fun?) had our bikes racked together and were issued consecutive numbers; I made a cursory look.

We all had details plaguing us. Rusty thought that he had left his packages of Gu - an easily-digestible gel, his food for the bike ride - back at the condo. There's so much to think of and organize on race morning! I had an extra Powerbar and gave it to him - he later discovered the packages of Gu in his biking shoe when he attempted to shove his foot in the shoe before the bike part of the race.

The swim, with more than 700 competitors, was a "mass start" in a narrow bay in waist-deep water. We were to "self-seed" ourselves, which means we were to determine how fast we could swim compared to others - that's hard to do, particularly for novices. I got somewhere in the middle, not out front with the fastest swimmers because I didn't want to be pushed under or have my goggles knocked off by someone faster coming from behind. When the horn sounded at 6:30 am, hundreds of pink and blue swim caps headed out to sea amid the cheers of hundreds of on-lookers. I tried to get a rhythm, but it was wild out there, with arms thrashing and feet kicking up a chop; I could see lots of lifeguards on surfboards and deep clear blue water. The sea was rough, full of swells; every time I came up for a breath or to look ahead I met a wave in the face!

I looked at the clock as I exited the water - forty-two minutes on my stopwatch - and scooted under the shower to rinse off the salt water and sand before running up the hill to put on socks and shoes, sunglasses, helmet, and the elastic belt showing my race number before jumping on my bike.

Melissa, who was leaning over a sawhorse around the transition area, yelled to me, "There are three in your age group in front of you, one with a twelve to fifteen minute lead. You can do it: go get 'em!" I knew that my swim hadn't been good, but that was a lot of time to make up, so it was a little demoralizing. I caught and passed two of them within the first forty-five minutes, and then I heard a friendly "You go, girl!" as Rusty came up beside me. We played leapfrog for the next two hours, making certain that we stayed at least three bike lengths apart to avoid a penalty for drafting by one of the many motorcycle judges on the course.

Gone were my fun imaginings along the Queen "K" Highway of the last few weeks; I didn't even notice the white-coral graffiti or look for the wandering donkeys. It was more important to concentrate on how I was feeling; I had swallowed a lot of ocean water and actually felt a little nauseous. The wind was vicious, drying the sweat before it could bead, leaving only a coating of salt behind; the volunteers at aid stations every nine miles had been coached in handing off bottles of water and

Gatorade to riders and did a wonderful job. As I rode back into town, I saw that I had averaged twenty miles an hour on the ride and felt good about that. I never saw the third woman out there in the lava fields.

A quick change to running shoes and a stop in the portajohn in transition put me in the direction of the "pit," a 4.4 mile "out-and-back," up one hill, down to a dead end and back up and over, without any hint of shade. I saw Ray jump out of the bushes - his portajohn - and we exchanged a "high-sign" and smiles. I felt good, squeezed some "tangerine Gu-with-double-caffeine" into my mouth along with some ice-cold water. Aid stations came every mile on the run, offering cold, wet sponges, ice water, Gatorade, and Coke; the volunteers were cheerful angels. I took most of the offerings to counteract the ninety-degree weather. The breeze off the ocean helped, and I felt good. I was actually having fun, gazed at the ocean and thanked God for giving me a body which could do this.

Passing Melissa as the run course looped back past the transition area, I heard her report, "The woman from Canada is ten to fifteen minutes ahead and doesn't look good. Go catch her!"

"What woman? What's her number?" I screamed back. Mary Ann and Gail were snapping pictures.

"#691!" - Melissa had been doing lots of investigating! And she was right; I finally saw #691 when she had passed the second turn around, and she did have about that much time on me. Melissa's only mistake was that she didn't "look bad"; she was not walking, and unless she were to walk, there was no way for me to catch her.

I saw Rob at an aid station, as he was heading back in to complete his race, chatting jovially with a volunteer; it was hard to be going away from the direction of the finish. Then I saw Rusty after I had made the final turn around. It was nourishing to me to see my friends, "the three R's", out there with me! But if I was reading the look on his face correctly, Rusty was struggling with the relentless sun; he's a big guy and doesn't dissipate heat easily.

The last three miles were not nearly as much fun, and the day became a mental game; "mind over matter" is truly a weak cliche' when applied to a mind which isn't computing things easily and a wornout body. My pace fell off some, but not much. I conjured up all kinds of comparisons to other three-mile runs I had done; I had several mantras I said over and over again, all psychologically positive in nature ("I love my feet ... I feel good ... only one more hill..."). It was not even like "heading to the barn" ... the finish line was more like the "Pearly Gates!" My time on the clock was five hours and twenty-nine minutes, about fifteen minutes faster than my goal! Ray and Rob were already done and our sweaty bodies hugged congratulations. The women were taking photos. We all waited expectantly for Rusty. I looked for snacks of protein and carbohydrates right away to begin the muscle-mending process.

My suspicions were soon confirmed when results were posted: #691, "Sandi from Vancouver, Wa.," was in fact fourteen minutes ahead of me at five hours fifteen minutes, breaking the course record by a large margin. Third place came in over six hours, more than thirty minutes behind me. My phone call to Nashville brought so many questions: "Could she possibly really be a man? Do you think she could have cheated?"

"No, she just really had an awesome race ... Sandi beat me fair and square." I had played the scenario over in my mind both ways. "I won the Ironman slot and began training for the event next October" - or the truth - I didn't win the slot.... Was I jealous? Absolutely! This may be the most difficult emotion to subdue.

In one way it was a loss; I had a solid chance out there. We encourage kids in sports because we say it teaches life's lessons; none of us is ever too old for life's lessons. Adults win and lose in life every day; we know that there are penalties for not following the rules, that with determination we can conquer seemingly insurmountable odds and that making excuses is not gracious. I had to keep reminding myself that this was a personal victory for me; I far exceeded my own goal and even took second place!

The awards banquet was delightful, out on the lawn beside the magnificent Pacific Ocean, relaxing on straw mats in the late afternoon with friends. We gathered for cocktails on the patio as the sun set and started talking about where we would go from here. Ray had won an Ironman slot in the lottery; he had finished third in his age group, but all he had to do today was to finish. He'll be training for that event in October. Thoughts of a July, 2001, trip to do the Vineman Triathlon in California were voiced; do the race (another one of the four Ironman qualifiers), then tour the wine country.... We were all interested.

Early the next morning I treated myself to one final indulgence; Leslie gave me a massage, using warm oil and island river stones. When we said good-bye, she gave me a hug and her Hawaiian blessing: "Malama Pono. Ke akua aloha pume oe," translating "Be in balance, with right thinking and right acting; may the God of love be with you."

What a wonderful journey it had been. I had done this for myself, with my family's blessings. My role as an athlete had required a disproportionate amount of my time for two months; it was time to regain balance and equilibrium. Still, I believe that if women don't do things for ourselves, we risk diluting two of the most important facets of our being - our strength as individuals and our ability to nurture others. I knew that the balance needed to be there as I returned home to wear my other hats: wife, mother, daughter, sister, homemaker, nurse practitioner. I would consider my career options, but, at the same time, I would certainly continue my training, which gives me the strength and the energy to maintain this balance of which Leslie spoke!

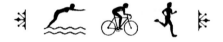

June 2000

>-I-◄►-O-◄►-I-◄

"The time you won your town the race,
We cheered you through the market place;
Man and boy stood cheering by,
And home we brought you shoulder high.
Today, the road all runners come,
Shoulder high we bring you home..."

A.E. Housman
To an Athlete Dying Young

"Can I come by and talk to you about your trip?" The call came within four hours of my arrival back home after being gone for five weeks. It was the writer of the "society" column for the local newspaper.

"Oh, sure, when do you want to come?"

"How about tomorrow afternoon? Don't worry, I know you have lots of dirty clothes piled up." Marilyn was savvy in knowing that if I thought about her request long enough I would decline.

In retrospect, I should have known better; a friend had mentioned that my results would be passed on to Kim, the woman who writes a weekly sports column on running for the paper. But Marilyn had called first. As it happened, I regretted not waiting for Kim, who would have put an entirely different spin on my whole adventure!

There I was, with not only my dirty clothes, five weeks worth of mail on the dining room table, Keith's junk from college blocking the entry hall, a house which needed cleaning, plus a terrible case of jet lag - but maybe more importantly, a yard which needed mowing and gardens which needed tending! For Marilyn is also considered the local gardening expert, somewhat of an authority on things green and flowering.

Actually, Marilyn wrote about what I had done and who I am in a fairly complimentary vein, but used adjectives such as "crazy" to describe my interest in doing these triathlons and the lifestyle I lead. She was curious about what she could do for her elevated blood pressure and extra weight, but didn't seem to pay much attention to my suggestions about aerobic exercise. Her final remark in the newspaper article emphasized that if she were I, she'd be heading out to work on the overgrown rose garden! My sister said the article was "tongue in cheek"; Keith said it was "ridiculous"; and friends said it was "cute." But my mother put it best. "She short-changed what you do."

Thinking about it a few weeks later, I realized that publicity such as this doesn't promote what active women are trying to accomplish; rather, it trivializes athletic accomplishment. Title IX, which mandated equality among male and female athletes at the university level (opponents claimed it was a radical plot to destroy football), was passed almost thirty years ago, but we are still experiencing gender disparity in the media and winning purses. Maybe my story got to the wrong woman!

It is a fact that many more women are becoming physically active, but we still have far to go. The aim of the International Triathlon Union Women's Committee is to provide information about issues to women around the world. Sport and sporting activities are important components of the culture of almost every nation, but in most places, females are not raised to be athletes and do not always have equity, despite Title IX in the USA. Also, women are traditionally more cautious, less likely to take risks, and less motivated to gain power; the characteristics of determination, confidence and aggressiveness have not been regarded as "feminine." Most women still grow up with the mentality that they should care for others before themselves.

The sport of triathlon is clean and healthy, and its future looks bright. It would be showcased to the world in the Olympics in September, 2000, in Sydney, where all would see a colorful, exciting event that has male and female participants. Hopefully, the media coverage would not portray triathlon as a grueling event focusing on competitors collapsing during and after competition.

Although it is important to have positive images from the media showing females participating in all sports, and I believe the triathlon in particular, images alone will not provide enough encouragement. We need a supportive environment which will attract women and girls and ensure their continued participation; and further, the notion that one needs to be a super athlete just to compete must be dispelled. Australia has the Females in Training (FIT) club for women of all ages and abilities who enjoy training in a non-competitive, supportive atmosphere. A Canadian friend of mine from the 1987 Ironman started a "women's-only" race in 1995 with 75 participants. Tina reported that 400 would compete this year! She was in the second year of providing a "how to" clinic which provides information, as well as encouragement. Endeavors such as these should result in a positive impact on the ratio of female participation in triathlon.

With an exercise program, one which doesn't take a lot of time, my newspaper interviewer friend could lower her blood pressure, raise her HDL (good) cholesterol and probably lose some weight. I wish she had come back in a few days; the house was straight, the clothes washed. And wow, the grass was mowed, and my roses were in glorious bloom! At any rate, it is becoming clear that participation in sport can enrich, enhance, and develop women's confidence, values, and attitudes, making them happier and more effective throughout their lives, whatever their roles may be.

>–⊦◄►–⊙–◄►⊦–◄

During the days after getting back home, I delivered gifts of t-shirts and hats from the World Championship race in Perth to my family, coaches and training buddies. I washed clothes, worked on my house and yard. Where would I go from there? Without a real goal ahead, it was easy to be bogged down by the stacks of bills and correspondence which had accumulated during the five weeks I had been gone. I was close to depression and felt like the new mother coming home from the hospital with a demanding infant. I had passed the culmination of many months of planning and training, and then such ordinary days followed.

I went for mediocre swims, short bike rides, slow runs ... but they were keeping me sane, just like exercise had kept me sane when the boys were little. Three boys under the age of five can cause all sorts of mental anguish; many times my sole chance for exercise had been to ride a stationary bike while they were napping or go for a run while Johnny was getting ready for work. Exercise back then had helped me get by without psychotherapy and Prozac, and it would help me again!

Bags were unpacked and repacked without ever getting to the attic. We had to get ready for Will's high school graduation in Vermont. I looked forward to one of my favorite runs in the northeast - a seven-mile loop which Johnny and I have done in the fall with red and gold leaves flickering in the branches of the birches and in the winter with snow and ice making the roads hazardous. Now, in the early summer, we would enjoy wildflowers and migrating songbirds as we traipsed through the hills.

I remember most places by mental pictures of where I ran there. I think of Chicago, and there's the windy run along Lake Michigan. San Francisco conjures images of running through the Golden Gate Park under the giant redwood trees. New York has me running through Central Park, beside rollerbladers and folks walking their dogs. When I think of Boston, I recall lovely brownstones along the course of the Boston Marathon, as well as burning legs. I think of peering up at the Eiffel Tower dressed in running clothes. Neighborhoods seem more intimate, even menus are better perused, as we travel on foot.

Virtually any woman of any age can start a walking, walk/run, and eventually running program. There are very few contraindications and so many rewards! It's the most time- and cost-effective exercise there is; the only requirements are a good pair of running shoes and some clothes for layering. I will run in any weather, anywhere. For a novice, one way to begin is to start with walking; then graduate to running between mailboxes or telephone poles. Running accomplishes more as a weight-bearing exercise for the prevention of osteoporosis - there is twice the impact of walking - and it gets the heart rate into the training zone for cardiovascular protection. In other words, you should be sweating.

Osteoporosis, a deforming and frequently fatal disease resulting from thinning of the bones, has received more of the attention it deserves in recent years. At least as many women will die from the complications of hip fractures as from breast cancer; the spine and wrist are the other bones most often affected. Many women find that as their "dowager's hump" becomes more pronounced and vertebrae fold down upon each other, there is less room for digesting food, and their clothes don't fit as well. A single, simple wrong move can lead to a very painful break. One's tendency to become osteoporotic depends 80% on heredity - did your mother or father have it? - and the other 20% is a result of adequate lifelong calcium (the primary mineral in bone) intake, largely through dairy products, exposure to estrogen, and weight-bearing exercise. Osteoporosis begins surreptitiously in many girls in their teenage and early adult years. Not having regular periods, indicating low estrogen exposure, not drinking milk or eating other dairy foods, and not exercising regularly are risk factors. Menopause and its declining hormone levels can accelerate bone loss, unless a women elects to take hormone therapy or one of the other anti-resorptive products, such as Fosamax, Actonel, or Evista. A bone density scan (Dual-energy X-ray Absorptiometry or DEXA) is an advisable screening tool for all menopausal women. See Appendix 4.

>-I-+>-O-<+-I-<

Will accepted his diploma on crutches, and he required lots of help packing up his belongings. Before flying home, we drove Keith to meet a friend who would help shuttle him up to Baxter State Park in Maine where he planned to start hiking the Appalachian Trail. The AT forms a line from north to south from the top of Mt. Katadin in Maine, over the highest mountains in the eastern United States, to the top of Springer Mountain in Georgia.

We were not completely supportive when Keith

began talking about taking a semester off from the University of Vermont to do this trek; a semester in England, Italy, or maybe even Nepal, would have given him college credit and be such a nice place to visit. But as time went on, his scheme took shape. He did the necessary research and purchased his own gear. The trail, marked by white blazes, is over 2,100 miles long and would take him five to six months. He planned to hike solo, take pictures, keep a journal, learn to play the harmonica. No plans were made as to when we would see him again; he wanted it that way. We said good-bye, took pictures, hugged a long time, and parted with tears in my eyes and fears of snakes and bears in my thoughts. He promised to call frequently when he stopped to resupply, take a shower, and wash clothes in towns along the way.

Will used the return portion of Keith's airline ticket (they look almost like twins on their picture ID's). We were a sight getting back home, with a bicycle box, ten pieces of luggage, and my elderly parents also in tow as we waited for delayed and rerouted airplanes.

Home for a week and off to a sports medicine meeting for Johnny in Sun Valley, Idaho. In the afternoons we rented mountain bikes and headed to trails in the hills. This sport is unique, different from riding a road bike. Most kids learn to ride bikes to cruise their neighborhoods. I remember my first bike with gears, a Kelly-green three-speed Raleigh with thinner tires. It made getting home from my friend's house a half mile away so much easier. Before that Christmas, I would ride down the hill, coasting most of the way with feet parallel to the ground, and either push the bike home or call for a ride. With the new bike, I could actually pedal back home, too! Bike riding is something that can be enjoyed again after many years of not riding; the mental pathways are still accessible with a little practice. As a form of exercise, it has the advantage of putting little strain on the joints and still has the benefits of being calorie-burning and weight-bearing.

Mountain bikes have fat tires with more tread to grip dirt and shock absorbers - but no motors! The technique needs to be practiced and some instruction is advisable (the sport was founded by adrenaline freaks). Benefits include getting back into scenery not available by car; you don't have to ride 60 miles per hour down cornices like the guys and girls at the Extreme Games. One afternoon Johnny and I joined a group of about ten riders; I was the token female. What a glorious three-hour ride up a two-lane dirt road to the top of a mountain. The washboard forced me to clench my teeth together to avoid biting my tongue. Moving through wet potholes, my feet at a high rpm to avoid being bogged down and putting my foot down in the water, I knew well that my back was becoming a brown canvas as mud was being thrown from the spokes of my rear wheel like the blades of a fan.

"Did you hear the thunder?" asked one of our companions, as we snacked on bananas and melted peppermint patties in our cheeks while reassembling at the top of the mountain. We didn't want to be caught out in an electrical storm in the mountains! Then two more riders in our group arrived and informed us that they had come around a corner right after a tremendous tree had fallen over the road. It was the fall of the tree, not a storm brewing, which we had heard.

The group followed "single-track," a narrow, smooth dirt path, through aspen forests, across shallow streams down the mountain for the next two hours; it was mountain biking at its best. Total concentration is required to avoid a "header" or "hugging a tree." I rode cautiously to avoid a wreck that day. As we descended, the path suddenly opened up into a breathtaking vista of the snow-crusted Sawtooth mountains; I dared not look too long or I would have forged a new and uncleared path through a meadow. I'll never think of Idaho without a mental image of hanging my "butt" over the back of my bike saddle, flying over rocks and down a mountain trail.

⊱┈⬩⟩⬩⚬⬩⟨⬩┈⊰

"Do you really still need that card?" I was back home and in the weight room at the gym. I had been doing a similar routine for almost a year now, and it was embarrassing that I had not committed to memory the order of the exercises, the seat heights and the approximate weights. A man older than I was calling my bluff; I would leave the card in the file next time and make myself do the exercises from memory.

Short-term memory loss is a common complaint voiced by "menopausals." Many "forgetful" women are worried that they are experiencing early signs of Alzheimer's, which is rarely the case. All of us have walked into a room in our house and wondered why we were there; remembering people's names is a big problem, as well. If you find yourself hanging up the dog, instead of the telephone, or can't remember your way home to where you've lived for many years, then see a doctor. Otherwise, practice mental exercises to keep the pathways healthy: balance the checkbook without a calculator, play bridge, do crossword puzzles, and concentrate on linking names with the letters of the alphabet or words that remind you of some characteristic of that person.

There is evidence to support taking regular vitamin supplements to pump up brain power, even though our primary sources of vitamins and minerals should be food and drink. The antioxidants scarf up "free radicals," those uncontrolled oxygen molecules which attack the cell walls of our muscles, brain, heart, and blood vessels. Unfortunately these scavengers are produced in greater quantities by the exercise we do to protect our hearts and bones. If we eat a healthy diet including lots of fresh fruits and vegetables, our bodies make antioxidants, but there are many convincing studies touting supplementation. My daily mishmash of supplements includes 500 mg. of Vitamin C, 400 IU of Vitamin E, a good multivitamin to provide the B vitamins, vitamins D and K, and trace minerals such as zinc, and a calcium supplement (to bring my daily total of elemental calcium up to 1200 mg. when the amounts in my diet are factored in). A few tips on calcium: The body can handle only about 500 mg at a time, so spread the consumption throughout the day. Calcium carbonate should be taken with meals or immediately after eating because it requires acid from digestion to be utilized; I prefer calcium citrate because it can be taken with or without food. Women ask about the need for additional iron and low-dose aspirin (81 mg) for cardiac protection. Athletes do lose iron through sweat, and young women may become anemic as a result of heavy menstrual periods. If fatigue is a problem, it is advisable to have a simple blood test for anemia before starting iron supplements, and of course there are other causes of fatigue, such as an underactive thyroid; taking too much iron can actually cause other problems. As for the aspirin, I have decided against it for now. I have no family history of heart disease, my exercise provides the best cardiovascular protection, and the gastrointestinal risks may outweigh potential benefits. (See Appendix 3).

I am not yet convinced by the claims for herbal supplements, even though sales represent billions of dollars a year. Lack of standardization and regulation may put the consumer at risk of getting little or no real active ingredient at the least, or pesticides and other toxic contaminants at the worst. The bottom line on "brainpower" is, again, exercise! We all need to exercise the neurons just like the quads.

>─┼─◄►─•─O─•─◄►─┼─◄

My Nashville buddies convinced me to drive over to do a triathlon in Chattanooga, Tennessee, two hours away, where they would join me from the Atlantic beach where they had been vacationing for the week. We met up the evening before the race, which was the state championship, and competed in the Olympic distance race on the banks of the Tennessee River. They claimed that they had been running and biking during the week, but not doing much swimming - another report of a shark attack on some kids swimming in the ocean on the east coast had discouraged them. It seemed to me that they were suffering the inevitable, unfortunate consequences of too much beach football and partying; Lyndell was "sick," Liz had to walk a large part of the ten kilometer run because of a pulled hamstring, and Debbie couldn't breathe after swallowing too much lake water! As Lyndell approached the finish line, George, Liz's husband, cheered from the sideline, "Good race, Lyndell!" She grunted back with a scowl on her sweaty, red face, "The only one having a good race is Emily."

I had beaten them all, which doesn't happen often - they are six years younger than I am and good athletes;

they skipped the awards ceremony and left for home. Only one other significant memory of the day remained. There were no bike racks; some competitors laid their bikes down. Because I use an open container with a straw between my handlebars for my Gatorade, I found a curb to keep the bike upright while propped on one of the pedals. I realized soon after starting the twenty-nine-mile ride that the bike must have turned over, spilling all of my liquid, and then someone had stood it back up. I'm sure that it was unintentional; luckily there were aid stations halfway through the course with full water bottles. There is a lot of trust and virtually no sabotage or poor sportsmanship in triathlon.

>–·–◆–·–○–·–◆–·–◁

Back at home while doing errands one afternoon in the car and listening to National Public Radio, I caught a blurb of an upcoming story about a triathlete named Judy. I knew instantly that I would be hearing about my friend Judy Flannery, who had been on the United States team with me at the World Championships at the Gold Coast of Australia in 1991. In 1997 she had been on a morning training ride on her bicycle in the countryside of Virginia with two friends. A car driven by a fifteen-year old without a driver's license, with the permission of his drunken father, crossed the center line and hit them head-on. The other riders were injured as they bounced up and over the sides of the car's hood, but Judy was killed.

Judy was one of those role models admired and emulated by many. Mother of five, frequent server to the homeless at soup kitchens in downtown Washington, DC, she was fiercely competitive in races. An inspiration, she had actually become faster in her fifties, winning the Triathlon and Duathlon World Championships for several years. Her daughter Erin had made a film "Judy's Time," commemorating her life.

Listening to the radio program about my friend, I was again reminded of the hazards which I often diminish when I ride my bicycle on the roads, as well as when I go running. I take obvious precautions, such as wearing a helmet, using a small rear view mirror to see what is approaching from behind, and strategizing appropriately; I avoid the busiest roads, and I abide by traffic laws. But the fact that many roads do not have a biking lane, or even a wide paved shoulder, contributes to the risk. I admit that I have had close calls, but I rationalize these, knowing that there are hazards in most endeavors we enjoy.

One day after swim practice, Rob said, "I've been carrying something for you around in my car, a memento of our trip from Ray, Rusty, and me." He handed me a clear plastic cylinder holding a grass-skirted, ukelele-playing, bronze-chested Hawaiian guy. He was immediately mounted on my dashboard. Every day as I turned a corner in the car, his green skirt swished in a sexy hula dance, even though his lips maintained a static grin, his lei didn't budge, and his fingers were stuck on the same strings. The response from the males on my homefront was dubious at best; they were embarrassed even thinking about reactions from friends and co-workers to the dancer, named "Ki" after my little Hawaiian hotel. Little by little they mellowed, however, and even enjoyed his movements, imagining what South Pacific tune he was strumming. Sometimes I imagined a wink and a dance of his feet in the shell-strewn sand under his toes.

My disappointment over not getting the slot for the Ironman was subsiding; I was having fun during the summer. I did not have to keep a tight, rigorous training schedule. Toward the end of June, a phone call came from the Triathlon Federation of America in Colorado Springs. "Would you reconsider the trip to Calais for the World Championship Duathlon?" asked Chad. He was putting together the American team for the race in France in early October. In March I had gone down to Birmingham, Alabama, to accept an award as Southeastern Triathlete of the Year in my age group and to do the Powerman Duathlon as training for the Perth and Kona races. Placing first at that race qualified me for the duathlon team, but I had passed up the offer, secretly hoping to be in Hawaii for the Ironman in October.

I demurred, "Can I think about it? I have barely unpacked my bags from the trip to Australia!" He said, "No problem, take your time," and offered to send me the literature concerning the event. The "duathlon" omits the swim portion of the triathlon, consists of a ten kilometer (6.2 mile) run, a sixty kilometer (36 mile) bike ride, and finishes with a five kilometer (3.1 mile) run. Swimming has always been my weakest leg, so this was a little tempting.... France in the fall would be nice.

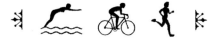

July 2000

>─┼─◆>─O─<◆─┼─<

*"The difference between a runner and
a jogger is an entry blank."*

Dr. George Sheehan

July the Fourth weekend found us with sixteen relatives up on the Cumberland Plateau in a cottage left by my grandmother to her seventeen grandchildren. Past vacations spent at the retreat were memorialized by hikes to mountaintops and swims in cold rivers; we've been lost on trails with no name and caught in forests after dark. In the last ten years, Johnny and I have habitually run a loop trail which takes a little over an hour to complete. One of my favorite runs in the world, it offers overlooks hundreds of feet into the valley below; breathing cool, fresh air, we talk little and scoot through tunnels of greenery and wildflowers. Our golden retriever Uta enjoys it just as much as we do. She actually loves running more than anything - except maybe "treats."

I love to run, too. Running requires little equipment; there is nothing to break, to lose, or to flat. It can become an out-of-body experience where one regains the carefree rhythm of childhood; my mind goes anywhere or nowhere at all. It gives me an escape, however briefly, from chores and obligations and clears my brain, helps me think clearly and creatively. I can plan with my mind and improve my body at the same time. Though considered eccentric by many people, running is becoming popular with more and more women as a way to achieve fitness. The history of women's running is short, really beginning in 1967, when gutsy Katherine Switzer dared to enter the Boston Marathon. She finished only by the grace of a body block delivered by her boyfriend to the race director Jock Semple, when he tried to tear off her race number upon discovering that K. Switzer was in fact a female! Women athletes everywhere thrilled when Joan Benoit Samuelson won the 1984 Olympic marathon gold medal - the first time women were allowed to run the marathon.

During almost twenty five years of running, I've never been bitten by a dog (a fistful of gravel is a good deterrent) or hit by a flying bottle thrown from the open window of a red pickup driven by a "redneck" (the two-fingered peace sign usually works when ignoring cat calls and whistles doesn't). My body language could be defined as "pleasant purpose," and I avoid deserted cemeteries, industrial areas, and big city parks in early morning runs if I'm alone.

A late night arrival to a strange place can be a cold, lonely experience, cured by an early morning jog. Xenophobias melt away as I run past a small boy, reminding me of my own three, and he pops one last "wheelie" on his skateboard, snaps it up under his arm and is swallowed up by a yellow school bus in the plains of Kansas. My own life energy improves as I glance over to see a group of elderly ladies and gentlemen strike a slow, synchronized posture in a morning session of Tai Chi, arms extended delicately, knees bent apart, eyes drinking in a red sun rising in the eastern sky over Chinatown in New York City. Fears evaporate as I run through a high mountain meadow, littered with multi-colored wildflowers, the grazing cows and their nursing calves parting to let me pass through them on a dirt road in the Colorado Rockies. I mumble, "It's OK, girls, don't be afraid," as much for me as for them.

My three pregnancies were fraught with bad varicose veins in my legs and feet, each pregnancy worse than the one before; the swollen vessels snaked up the tops of my feet and ankles where they bulged a dark purple, and they throbbed. Heavy support hose had to be pulled on before I got out of the bed in the morning - ugly, to be sure, but they reduced the pain. I remember sitting beside the swimming pool on hot summer days in the south, wearing the stockings, sweat running down my swimsuit. Running has definitely improved my circulation; the veins are less noticeable, although I know they're there. One Saturday morning Johnny and I stopped to pick up some bagel sandwiches after a run in the park, still dressed in shorts and t-shirts. I took the bag from the counter and before I turned around (so the woman standing behind me hadn't seen the "crows feet" around my eyes nor the smile lines at the corners of my mouth), the words were said, "You have beautiful legs ... runners' legs." I figured she was talking to someone else - I'd never received a compliment like that - I could hardly utter the "thank you."

Many women prefer relaxed, uncompetitive runs; but entering a race keeps one motivated to run and exercise. A race calls attention to nutrition, stretching, and realistic goals. Being among other women who are competing and are strong is contagious, spreading emotional resilience, strength, and courage. This is a healthy habit at any age.

I told myself all these things when I signed up for the Firecracker 5K on July 4th. Not a long distance, but in the heat and humidity of the south even 3.1 miles can be quite uncomfortable. The shade was sparse, and lots of people got overheated. I tolerate the heat better than most, though I don't like it. My twenty-one minute fifty-six second time put me first in my age group; the 7:04

minute-per-mile pace wasn't bad in those conditions. I was happy with the effort. Additionally, I could more easily rationalize those baked beans, potato chips, and fudge cake I planned to eat later that day!

My narcissistic existence got a break! My sister had orchestrated a trip for us to take our eighty-one-year-old mother to visit her three older siblings in Tacoma, Washington. To be honest, I was not excited about this, as I conjured up thoughts of escorting them with their canes up ramps into restaurants where they would talk too loudly because their hearing aids were chirping like birds and tell stories over and over again because they couldn't remember that they had told them before. I imagined that my nights would not be restful because I'd be sharing a room with my mother who makes multiple nocturnal trips to the bathroom and turns on the light at ungodly hours. It turned out to be quite a fun time, seeing cousins I knew as a small child and visiting the clear lake where my eighty-eight-year old Uncle Billy taught me to water ski when I was a young girl. We took a day off to let the older generation reminisce and took my niece to hike at Mt. Rainier.

Rainier, seventy-five miles east of Tacoma, in the Cascade mountains, is the second tallest mountain in the lower forty-eight states. (At 14,495 feet, Mt. Whitney in California is actually eighty-five feet higher.) Rising out of the Paradise Valley, the mountain is comprised of twenty-six glaciers which feed swift streams and tumbling waterfalls that roar through the valleys below. Each year 9,000 to 10,000 hardy souls attempt to reach the summit of Rainier, but only half succeed. The full ascent from timber line to the summit is more than 9,000 feet, making it the longest in the lower forty-eight states - that is what makes the endeavor so physically demanding. My great uncle was a climber of the western peaks, as was my uncle. Every year Uncle Billy asked me when I was going to climb "the mountain."

Johnny and I hatched a deal when the boys were three, five, and seven years old. "If you and Aunt Mary Louise will keep the boys, we'll climb the mountain." Having no children of his own, Uncle Billy has doted on his many nieces, nephews, and now great nieces and great nephews; the children love being with their fun, jovial uncle. (My Will was born on his birthday and is named for him). We made the climb as part of a Rainier Mountaineering Incorporated (RMI) guided group. They are a superb outfit of experienced guides, including lots of Everest veterans. I was the only female in the group to summit in 1983; one woman elected not to continue and waited in a sleeping bag on the mountain until we were on the way down.

The Rainier climb is a three-day commitment. The first day involves learning the techniques of climbing as a member of a roped team, self-arrest with an ice ax, rest-step climbing, and pressure breathing, as well as proving to the guides that you're strong enough to not hold the group back. The second day is a long, slow hike from the lodge at Paradise at 5,000 feet across the snow fields to a hut at Camp Muir, at about 10,000 feet. After a meal and a few hours of "sleep" on a three-tiered wooden shelf in the hut, the guides determine if the weather looks promising for an assault on the summit. If it's a "go," you gobble some oatmeal and hot chocolate, put crampons on your boots, don your helmet and headlamp (it's one or two in the morning), rope up with a team of three or four climbers and one guide, and the entire group of four to five teams strikes out across the glacier.

The ribbon of light on the snow from the headlamps illuminates the night and moves up around

Disappointment Cleaver and over numerous crevasses under a heavy canopy of still and shooting stars. The summit, at 14,410 feet, is usually attained around sunrise; the view through the thin air is crisp and ethereal, as the other mountain peaks of St. Helens (what remains after the explosive eruption of 1985 which killed sixty people and blasted more than 1,000 feet from the peak of the mountain), Hood, and Baker and the burning sun pierce the hazy dawn. Signing the register at the top, near where the dormant volcano still spews gassy fumes from its cone, leaves proof that you were there. The third day ends with descending all the way to Paradise. It is an exhausting three days!

Johnny decided to take each of our three boys to climb the mountain when he turned fifteen, as kind of a rite of passage. During Will's climbing year my two brothers and I went, also - as did Keith - because his year the group had been forced to turn around without summitting due to driving sleet and wind. I had not planned to do this adventure again, but just could not stand the thought of so many of my family being up there on that mountain without me! I'll never forget looking over by the light of my headlamp in the middle of the night, with a mother's special interest and alarm, when I heard one of the guides tell Will, "You have your crampons on the wrong feet!" The crampons, which fit over the hard, plastic climbing boots, must be strapped in a crisscross fashion over and behind the ankles and buckle on the outside of the feet; Will's were buckled on the inside of his ankles, a potential cause of tripping. We were in a rush to leave Camp Muir for the summit. "It won't matter on the way up - you can change them on the top," the guide said with authority. I must admit that I worried about that for the next six hours as we trudged up the glacier in the dark. Everest may be the "roof of the world," but we felt we were certainly in the attic when we attained the top; adrenalin ricocheted among the six of us who were related. There was a brief rest period; Will used most of the time methodically fixing his crampons - everything takes longer at that altitude. We snacked and took pictures. Our guides hurried us to start the trek down the mountain; they don't want to be caught too high up when the sun begins to melt the ice cap, opening up dangerous, new crevasses. I was tiring and wasn't picking my feet up. One of the sharp metal picks of my right crampon caught the strap around the left ankle, and I fell hard, my kneecap striking directly on a rock. I hobbled into Camp Muir. Johnny determined that there didn't appear to be any significant injury, most likely just a bad bruise. At any rate, the heaviest contents of my backpack were divided among my family members, taking some of the load off of my injured knee. When we finished the climb and called my mother from the guide center at Paradise, as requested, to let her know we were safe at the bottom, she was so relieved. Every year or two, climbers fall into the crevasses or are suffocated under avalanches. There have been at least ninety-three climbing-related deaths on the mountain since record keeping began in 1887. The worst accident in American climbing history occurred in 1981 when eleven climbers were killed in an ice fall, some buried under ice chunks the size of houses, others careening thousands of feet on the glacier.

Our summit climb in 1997 included two female guides (and three other female climbers). "Would you like to be part of an all-female team to climb Denali (the highest peak in Alaska) next summer?" asked one of the guides. I took this as a tremendous compliment, but deferred. It was a thrill to accomplish the Rainier climb with so many members of my family, but I was not sure if I planned to do it again, much less a three-week trek to Alaska! It's not the physical challenge that deters me, but the terribly frightening views of bottomless crevasses as one takes thousands of small, methodical steps at just the right pace not to cause too much or too little slack in the rope for the team. Johnny vows he will celebrate his sixtieth birthday with another climb - I need to work on my vertical foot lift if I plan to go along! Jumping rope and Pilates classes might help.

⪼━┥◆⟩━○━⟨◆┝━⪻

One hot and humid Saturday morning in July I almost lost our best running companion; to be honest I almost killed her. Uta was a three-year old golden retriever, our third golden. Mariah was first; she ran like the wind. Then there was Greta, named after the lanky, blond Swede who won the Olympic gold in the marathon. Greta didn't live up to her running potential because of a pelvic fracture sustained as a pup when she slid on the ice under the garbage truck. Uta was named after the German woman who won the one-hundredth Boston Marathon. I was far behind her in that race in 1996. My family watched in awe as Uta Pippig approached the finish line, blood and diarrhea streaming down her legs. She was oblivious to any problem, so strong and determined; our pup would live up to that legacy.

And she did. When we run four miles, she'll go eight; if it's ten for us, she probably puts in twice the distance. She chases squirrels and deer and will try to rout out any creature from its hideout. She knows when we put on running shoes that there's a chance she can go; she is one hundred percent enthusiastic no matter what the weather.

Summer runs in the south can be dehydrating, so we carry a water source and a ziplock bag to allow for Uta to drink, too. Percy Warner Park, with 2,058 acres, is a few miles from our house. With over thirty miles of nicely shaded roads and trails, it is one of the largest such parks within city limits in the country.

I planned to do the 11.2 mile loop that day; it was just Uta and me, because Johnny and Will were on a college orientation trip to Western Washington University. My running mileage needed to be increased a bit as we had decided to make the trip to Calais, France, in early October for the world championship duathlon.

It was hot; after the first few miles Uta lost her usual excitement over exploration in the woods and stuck right by my side. I stopped every couple of miles for water breaks; at mile seven, we took advantage of the hose at the golf course to drink all we wanted. We stopped at a picnic table by the road at mile nine to drink, rest, and walk up the next hill. Uta began to lag behind, looking for any cool place to lie down; I coaxed her on. With only one-fourth mile to go, she stopped at the back of a parked car, hoping it was ours, then collapsed on the ground and couldn't get up. I knew she was in trouble and tried to carry her, but her sixty five pounds were too heavy a load for me. A car came by and the driver took us down the hill to my car. With my flashers blinking I sped to my veterinary clinic, wondering as I drove if they would be open at 12:15 on a Saturday (I discovered that they usually close at noon but had been busy and hadn't locked the doors). I could see in my rearview mirror that Uta was limp, though breathing.

I ran into the clinic with my story of panic, they yelled "Stat." A big man came out and carried Uta in; Dr. Bell, Carla and Daniel started to work. They covered her with ice packs and wet towels and got an IV started. She was carried to a cool tub to get her temperature down and then started on plasma and antibiotics. Sampson, a large sweet mixed breed with big brown eyes, donated whole blood; Dr. Bell felt this might give her a better chance to battle the blood clotting which is the usual cause of death in heat exhaustion. Another vet in the office wandered in, saw the small red spots called peticiae on her inner thighs, and muttered, "that's a bad sign."

I felt enormous guilt; how could I have done this to her? She has total trust and always wants to please. I had ignored her signals. I was far too determined to stick to my plan, too hard-headed, inflexible. If only I had taken a short cut back to the car before she got into trouble.... if she died, how could I break the news to Johnny and the boys?

Uta was brought back to the exam table and covered with warm blankets to elevate her internal temperature to normal. I kept rubbing her, whispering her name in her ear, talking to her as she lay limp. I was praying to the God of pets and people. Suddenly she looked at me with recognition; I was thrilled by this sign of improvement! More rubbing and talking. When her tail started wagging, slapping against the table, I shouted out loud and hugged her hard.

Dr. Bell wanted to keep her there for the afternoon on the IV and then transfer her to the emergency pet facility for the night, since their clinic is closed on weekend nights. "She's not out of the woods. Her kidneys or her liver can be affected," he emphasized. I left to shower and pray some more.

The transfer to the emergency clinic and more vets made it necessary for me to try to explain again how I could have let this happen; such stupidity is inexcusable. I don't know why, but everyone was very kind to me, and said I could call at any hour to check on her.

DIC, "dead in cage," is the vets' acronym to describe the condition of disseminated intravascular coagulation which results from heat exhaustion and is usually fatal (this condition can be deadly for people, too).

All afternoon and night I moped and was haunted by the vision of this sweet, fit dog being put through hell by her "caring" master. I didn't want to talk to anyone. But, wouldn't you know it, Johnny, Will, and Keith all called home, and I had to confess. A few words of empathy kept me from complete self-flagellation. Keith said, "Mom, it could have been me; I took her running many times this summer when I didn't know if she'd make it or not." I suppose we were all learning a horrible lesson.

When I awoke at 4:30 am Sunday morning and called the clinic, she was still stable, though her temperature was a little low. As the day wore on, her condition improved, and I was able to bring her home. She was spoiled for weeks, even allowed to sleep on the bed. I've heard many stories of similar occurrences since this happened, with mostly bad outcomes for the dogs. She would be more susceptible to the heat after this near-death episode, so we would have to be extra careful with her running from then on.

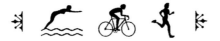

August 2000

"Keep close to Nature's heart ...
Climb a mountain or spend a week in the woods."

John Muir

Two weeks had passed since we had last heard from Keith. He had been thoughtful about checking in with us, leaving messages on the answering machine if we were not at home, stating where he was along his sojourn. We were relieved that he had survived the "hundred mile wilderness" where there is literally no access to the outside world. He had continued to pare down his backpack, mailing back items which had seemed essential two months ago but became superfluous weight. I found that I was lying awake at night worrying about him. When I was a child, the monsters were under the bed; since I've been an adult, the monsters seem to be in my head!

Insomnia is an affliction unbelievably common among the menopausal women I see in my practice. Sleep efficiency, the amount of time one actually spends asleep when in bed, declines steadily throughout life. The inability to sleep may be caused by worry over life's travails; sometimes night sweats are the culprit. Often, though, it is a developed pattern, maybe rooted in years of keeping an ear alert for a baby or a teenager out too late. It becomes a habit, one all too familiar to me. Fall easily and deeply asleep, only to awaken in a few hours to toss and turn. I've balanced my checkbook, unloaded

93

the dishwasher, even cooked at two and three in the morning. A good night's sleep (seven to eight hours) can become an elusive struggle.

I have learned through experience that nothing produces the "recovery" of a natural sleep better than falling asleep naturally. Sleep aids of many kinds, over the counter as well as prescription, interfere with the different stages of sleep architecture and result in "rebound" insomnia or a drugged feeling well into the next day. That said, there are situations in every woman's life when fatigue can become chronic from sleep deprivation; at those times coping skills suffer and even immunity may be reduced. Prescription sleeping medicine is the best and most reasonable option then. Hormones (estrogen and progesterone) are said to be helpful. Though I take hormones myself, I find these claims not totally substantiated scientifically, largely anecdotal.

The best advice I've gotten and pass along to patients is similar to the old one we were given as children - count sheep. Well, not really. Worthwhile suggestions include avoiding caffeine and exercise before bed, keeping the bedroom cool, and reserving the bed for sleep and sex; take only small (thirty minutes max) "naps," when necessary. Ovaltine mixed with warm milk or "Sleepytime tea" are good bedtime or middle-of-the-night snacks. Learning to relax, one tiny muscle at a time, head to toe, then picturing your "mind's eye" or a broom sweeping worries away has worked for me as well as anything. Those times when nothing works, and I've really slept only a few hours, exercise actually makes me feel much better. Endorphins, the body's natural pain killers, are a byproduct of exercise and keep me going the rest of the day.

I decided to call Keith's bank to find out if he had been using his debit card and, thereby, I would know at least that he was alive.

"I am sorry, but you are not listed on his account, and I cannot give you any information," the teller said over the phone.

I requested a conversation with a bank officer and gave her a sob story. "I really don't want to know how much money he has in his account, only that he has been using the card. I'm so worried that he has been hurt and am considering calling the FBI department of missing persons."

She laughed, was silent for a brief time, and then said, "Don't worry, I really think that he is just fine." Her tone was reassuring (she probably saw on the computer that he was using the card), and I hung up. It wasn't thirty minutes later that the phone rang; it was Keith, calling from a small town in Pennsylvania.

He had covered more than six hundred miles in seven weeks and was emotionally very positive with his experience. Our oldest son Johnny was in school in New York City and had driven over to spend one night on the trail with him. They had hiked up to the top of a ridge, Johnny with his guitar. They shared a special night for brothers, playing music and talking late, I'm sure.

Keith told me with excitement of seeing a large timber rattlesnake in New Jersey; he had hiked within a few feet of the snake before seeing it. I had been mailing care packages every week or two to the post office in towns he planned to visit along the trail. Usually it was necessary for him to hitch-hike a ride into town, because the trail would cross the highway a few miles out. I heard about one very special lift.

"Put on the helmet and jump on," demanded the deep voice of the woman driving the motorcycle with the sidecar. With his fifty-pound pack resting in his lap it was the ultimate ride; he admitted that he wished some of his fellow hikers had seen him then!

"Thru-hikers," as those hardy souls undertaking the entire trail are called, adopt a trail name which follows them in a network, as they sign registers at different shelters and word of mouth passes stories and identities along. He told me about "Looking Glass," "Hypothetical," "Not there yet," "Nimble Ned." Keith was "Old Man Sam" ... "Sam" for short. His first name is Samuel.

"I'd better go, I'm supposed to be somewhere," I said after the conversation had gone on for over thirty minutes.

"Please don't hang up, I've got so much more to tell you." These words were music to a mother's ears; I was late to wherever I was going.

>─┤─◆⟩─⚬─⟨◆─┤─<

Thursday mornings on hot summer days found four or five of us "girls" heading out regularly into the countryside, chatting as we rode. We were usually able to adjust work schedules to accommodate the time. The long rides would last anywhere from two to five or six hours, plenty of time to talk about many topics with few verboten subjects.

Becky was our mechanic, assisting us with changing tires when the need arose, as well as our authority on the latest internet and published information on exercise. Lyndell would inform us about the bacteria she was culturing in the lab, Liz would give us pointers on the fine elements of golfing and what was happening in the realm of professional sports, and I would entertain them with stories of patients, as well as educate them about what different tests women were advised to get at different ages.

The idea of yearly PAP smears, mammograms, and bone density screening was all fine and good, but when I got to the tests to detect colon cancers, they, like most people, were squeamish. I reminded them that colon cancer is one of those silent cancers and is often found only after it has spread to other parts of the body. The American Cancer Society recommends that a baseline sigmoidoscopy be done at the age of 50, and, if clear, at five year intervals, with a colonoscopy, which investigates further up the colon, at ten year intervals.

"When you turn 50, not long from now you know, you need to follow my example." And so I entertained them one morning telling them about Johnny's and my recent experience.

We had decided to go straight for the colonoscopy to get a more thorough report and elected to submit to the humiliating experience on the same day, back to back (not literally!) with the same doctor, in order not to spoil more than one 24-hour period with the necessary diet restrictions. After a 12-hour liquid diet of jello and beef broth, we began the appointed day with a nice run in the park. Then the nasty preparation began. We were each to drink a gallon of the prescribed liquid (ghastly in taste) which would clean out our guts over the course of two hours. We each disappeared with jugs, books, magazines, and cell phones into our individual bathrooms. A wise friend had recommended to just "stay put" and not to try leaving the toilet to do other things (your rear end just gets raw from wiping!) Periodically we would ring one another up to compare notes as to the other's progress on the level in the jug.

The test itself wasn't bad. Anesthetized just enough to lose all inhibitions, I watched the monitor with interest as the long tubing searched up my lower gastrointestinal track. My report was clean, but Johnny had a couple of polyps which were removed during the procedure. These polyps can become cancer, so it was recommended that he return for the test again in three years as follow-up. The good news was that the polyps were found; the bad news was that he wouldn't have me to commiserate with him in the next bathroom three years from that time! My sweet sister Susie drove us home, stopping long enough for us to pick up a nice steak and a bottle of wine.

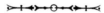

Johnny and I flew to Colorado to take a course in wilderness medicine; the brochure had been enticing us for years. There were workshops geared to assembling a first-aid kit of travel medicine, as well as practical instructions on what to do in the event of being lost in the wild (take a whistle and a large plastic bag to use as emergency shelter and learn to use a signal mirror). We were taught the basics of recognizing avalanche danger, how to treat altitude sickness, scuba diving injuries, and snake bites. I learned that males are actually more susceptible to high altitude illness than females.

We became familiar with the concept of "live high, train and race low," the theory being that the increase in red blood cells resulting from the body's natural response at higher elevations provides extra oxygen to working muscles when training at sea level. This is the theory behind sleeping in the hypobaric chambers used by some of our elite athletes. I never stayed in the mountains long enough to become truly altitude-adjusted or to benefit from the extra red blood cells; all our runs were "slogs" (slow jogs) because we were gasping for air.

I attended a special session for women in the wilderness, addressing our unique needs. The topic of the female's menstrual cycles provided some interesting discussions. "Pack out everything that you take in" is a rule with special meaning for a woman having her period in the wilderness. No one seemed to have the answer to the question of whether the odor of human blood produced by a woman who is currently bleeding and/or has soiled sanitary products in ziplock bags in her backpack would attract wild animals. This is one thing that I certainly don't miss about menopause!

The idea of being able to skip periods altogether with the use of oral contraceptives (oc's), where the week of placebos and therefore the withdrawal bleed are omitted, was appealing to many women. There don't appear to be any side effects to this approach. For women between the ages of 40 and 50 when fluctuating hormone levels can lead to irregular, heavy, and prolonged periods and unexpected bleeding, low-dose oc's are a reasonable option. Those years are called the peri-menopause. Normally the monthly cycles eventually become lighter and further apart, ultimately stopping altogether. Women are in menopause when they have had a year without menstrual bleeding. The average age is 51 and has been for centuries. What a great time to start camping!

This was another wonderful trip, included some beautiful runs and a hike to Buckskin Pass, at 12,000 feet, but lingering in the back of my mind was my repeat diagnostic mammogram scheduled for the end of the month.

I had followed the recommendation of the American Cancer Society to begin annual screening mammograms at the age of 40. Finding breast cancer early makes treatment much easier and increases survival rate. I've had to return for additional films called spot compression views and ultrasound several times during the last three years. There is a dense area with microcalcifications in my right breast which the radiologists continue to study for any increase in number or change in size because a small number of such calcifications may represent early breast cancer. These calcifications are not thought to have anything to do with diet or calcium supplements, usually represent changes that occur as a result of aging, and are found in most women over the age of forty. In addition, breast density changes with age, weight gain and loss, and as a result of oral contraceptives and hormone replacement. Most cancers in the breast are actually found by women themselves; however, the area of concern in my breast cannot be felt.

Like most women, I have friends and acquaintances who have breast cancer, and I feared such a diagnosis. Breast cancer is one of the most common cancers in women; yet I read recently in the medical literature that women in a study by the National Cancer Institute tremendously overestimate their risk of getting and dying from breast cancer, thinking it was twenty-five times higher than it actually was. In fact, less than five percent of U.S. women will die from breast cancer, whereas about fifty percent will die from cardiovascular disease (heart attack and stroke). The fact that one in every eight women will get breast cancer is true, but it's only true for those women who live to the age of ninety (only one in twenty women get it before age fifty).

There are so many myths which surround the use of hormones, and their effect on one's risk of breast cancer; simply stated, hormones do not cause cancer. Tons of dialogue on what is natural floods the press. To set the record straight, the female sex hormones of estrogen, progesterone, and testosterone are produced naturally by a woman's body until she reaches menopause, when these hormones fall off dramatically. Until the mid-1900s, women lived only a few years after "the change." Women are now living much longer and are attempting to replicate the body's natural exposure to female hormones.

The reduced hormone levels of the postmenopausal stage affect the entire body, often resulting in distinctive, disturbing symptoms. And, while this is not a disease state requiring medical intervention, postmenopausal women are at greater risk for developing many conditions associated with aging. Hence the option of hormone replacement therapy (HRT), as well as proliferating nontraditional remedies such as herbs. Recent research indicates that the yearly increase in breast cancer risk for women taking hormone replacement therapy (HRT) was two percent, close to the same as the natural increase in risk that women face simply by getting older. Many of the hormones are made from natural products, such as soybeans and yams. Those women who elect to take HRT and do get breast cancer appear to have higher rates of survival. Of course, every woman must weigh her own risks and decide for herself, as we wait for more research. (See Appendix 4)

>-+-+)-+-O-+<+-+-<

I made the decision to go to Calais, France, for the duathlon in early October and began training with a heart-rate monitor. I had won the tool at the Powerman Duathlon qualifying race in Alabama back in the spring. I wanted to learn to sustain my heart rate longer during the stress of a race without becoming fatigued;

this gadget provided a window into my body's physiology. The heart rate represents the effects of exercise on the entire body, particularly the heart, lungs, and muscles. Basically, the harder the workout, the faster the heartbeat.

The method of determining one's heart rate used to be to stop exercising long enough to feel with two fingers for the pulse over the carotid artery at the neck and count the beats for a minute. The new monitors, consisting of a transmitter that Velcros around the rib cage and a receiver worn like a wristwatch, now provide portable biofeedback with the accuracy of a hospital EKG. Some sportsbras have a special pocket for the transmitter, though I do not use one. Wearing the contraption was like having a coach providing constant feedback. Easy to use, the electrodes sense your heart rate on the chest, do the calculation and display it while exercising.

The first step was to determine my Maximum Heart Rate (MHR) because the science of exercising in a "training zone" is based on a percentage of MHR. Exercising at too high an intensity too often is not necessary and can, in fact, lead to injury and burnout. But I knew I needed to occasionally push myself a bit uncomfortably, especially when I went for weeks without doing a race of any kind.

There are several formulas for arriving at one's MHR, other than the "run-hard, throw-up" way. The most common formula is to subtract your age from 220; another one is to take 205 minus half your age. Still another formula is to take 210 minus half your age in years, minus five percent of your body weight in pounds, plus four for men and zero for women. Whatever the formula, take the average and remember that there is a significant margin of error in each formula and that age, as well as present level of fitness, makes a difference! Beginners find that the positive feedback provided by using a monitor tells them that their heart rate will be lower with the same workout over time and that they get stronger with regular exercise.

Different "zones" are derived by taking 50% to 90% of the MHR in 10% increments. Light exercise can be as little as 50% of the MHR for the beginner and can be beneficial to the heart, lungs, and muscles. To lose weight/burn fat and build fitness gradually, one should exercise at 60%-70% of the MHR. I could maintain my aerobic base by going out comfortably and chatting all the while at 70% to 80% of my MHR. To maintain excellent fitness condition and get ready for Calais I needed to go 80% to 90% some of the time.

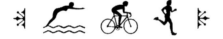

September 2000

"A newspaper wrote that I was too old.
It made me so mad that I went out and won four golds."

Fanny Blankers-Koen
Sprinter from the Netherlands
who was 30 when she won four
events in the 1948 Olympics.

This was the month of the Music City Triathlon, and "the girls" were making many bicycle rides on the race course, allowing for lengthy conversations. "Becky has been reading about an interesting aspect of cycling," Lyndell said to me with a straight face when we commenced the next outing. "It seems that twenty percent of females have had an orgasm while riding."

Liz continued. "Since you weren't here last week, the four of us decided you must be the necessary missing piece of data to fulfill the statistics." Everyone laughed; there followed a pregnant pause as all sunglasses panned in my direction.

My immediate response was an explanation of the requirements of scientific research and a question of the reliability and validity of Becky's study. "So, Becky, how many women were in this study? Was there a control group? What kind of bikes were they riding?" I was dodging the obvious question! After three hours of sweating together, I assured them that our population did not support the findings of Becky's study.

The Music City course is one of the hilliest and most difficult anywhere. The late summer morning was rainy when I responded to my alarm clock, but the weather did not dissuade many of the 400+ entrants. As the swim began, the precipitation quit. The water was cool enough to allow wetsuits, the buoyancy providing an equalizing factor for those of us who are not as fast in the water.

Lyndell and Liz are in the age group below me, so we are in different categories for winning awards. We are friendly competitors, but in a race we do race each other. At the end of the mile swim the three of us were assisted up the slimy, algae-covered boat ramp within a mere five seconds of one another to cheers and clapping! All of my swimming with coach Carol had paid off. Yanking off our wetsuits, pulling on our bike shoes, and snapping the straps of our helmets were quickly accomplished; they gained a few seconds on me in transition.

Unfortunately the roads were still wet, and there were numerous bike wrecks. One of the casualties was Liz, who went down as she rounded a corner; she got back on her bike and continued the race at a slower, achy pace. "How bad do I look?" she asked as I came up to her on my bike.

I could see her raw, red leg and shoulder, a bad case of "road rash." "You're bleeding," I replied, "but I don't think you need any stitches." She encouraged me to go on.

Soon enough I was off the bike, had switched shoes, and was back out on the course for a run in the hills. I couldn't ignore a "stitch" in my side as water sloshed around in my stomach and distracted my concentration. This is a common and annoying complaint to new runners, and no one really knows the cause. I couldn't catch Lyndell, who was not far ahead of me when we finished the bike leg. She saw me and the look on my face (which divulged my discomfort) as she completed the turn-around of the run and shouted, "I'll slow down when you pass me." Some kind of strategy and sense of humor.

Johnny and Will had come out to photograph the event. My finish-line pictures are usually not to my liking because there's such a pained look on my face. I decided to smile as I approached the final stretch despite how badly I was feeling. I am so happy I did that because I liked my pictures for the first time and resolved to look ecstatic for finish line photos from then on. Smiling doesn't make the discomfort any worse or any better! Lyndell finished second female overall, and I was tenth in a field of over 90; the other eight girls were young enough to be our daughters! I won the Masters division, comprised of those over forty.

Friends informed us that Jim Ward, a legendary age-group triathlete, had died of an apparent heart attack while on a training ride on September 4th. Johnny and I remember well when Jim bounced effortlessly off the podium three feet above the beach after accepting his award at the Gulf Coast Half-Ironman distance race in Florida two years before; he had moved like a much younger man. At 83 years he was still competing, having completed the Hawaiian Ironman at age 77. He had become an ambassador for the sport and appeared on ABC's "Good Morning America." Jim was a good friend and competitor of our local hero, John Hazen, who at 84 was still going out for long bike rides with us in the country and doing trail work for the Sierra Club. Individuals like Jim and John are constant reminders that we never have to grow "old" just because the numbers say so and that we can achieve so much when we just allow ourselves to try. They provide real life proof that an active lifestyle may relate to one's longevity and quality of life more than any other factor. Recent research in fact shows that keeping the heart, lungs, and muscles fit can stave off frailty and that inactivity is a strong predictor of premature death.

>━┥━◄►━━O━◄►━┥━◄

This was the month of the 2000 Summer Olympics in Sydney, Australia, where the sport of triathlon made its global debut; as a "spectator event" the first year, it would be considered as a repeat sport in future games. The women's race was the opening event from "downunder." My training buddies came over to share dinner and watch the media coverage. It was exciting, and we felt that it was well-reported.

Triathlon has grown quietly over its quarter-century life, but this was a dramatic introduction to the world. The sport may have come of age as the 48 women dived from a platform below the Opera House into Sydney Harbor. Divers bobbed beneath the bay with shark-discouraging devices, and an armada of attendants on surfboards protected them from above as luxury yachts and schooners enjoyed the splashing spectacle. The 200,000-odd spectators who lined the bike and run courses four deep on the streets around the Royal Botanic Gardens were not disappointed!

My friends and I knew how hard these women had worked. We go there in our dreams... when we "grew up," we would be professional triathletes, not "age-groupers." If we were thirty or forty years younger, I know we would have aspired to be one of the three women representing the USA in the triathlon.

Sheila Taormina, who won a gold medal in swimming in the summer Olympics in Atlanta in 1996, began training in this new combination of skill sets and led the swim segment by an incredible thirty-six seconds. Jennifer Gutierrez showed strength and bravado when she and a German competitor made repeated break-aways on the bicycle, once again putting an American in the lead, only to be sucked up by the pack in the draft-legal race. Our third American, Joanna Zeiger, stayed with the leaders and placed an honorable fourth at the end of the race. Carol Montgomery, a Canadian running machine, tragically crashed in a threesome, taking her out of the triathlon, as well as the women's 10,000-meter run later in the week. Someone's dreams were broken in an instant, and it was terrible; another's were actualized just as quickly before the global audience.

The real race boiled down to the final 5k of the 10k run. Aussie-favorite Michellie Jones had beaten Brigitte McMahon from Switzerland in the Sydney World Cup, a dress rehearsal held in April. We all know there are no guarantees in the Olympics, but there was no reason to think this race would end any other way, especially with Michellie running for thousands of supporters on her home turf who were chanting "Aussie, Aussie, Aussie, Oi, Oi, Oi." Michellie never gave up; she ran her heart out. But Brigitte had rehearsed the sprint finish in numerous practice sessions, visualizing the Aussie behind her. She pulled ahead in a deadly kick, her strat-egy delivering her a gold medal and the immense pride of her husband; her infant daughter would someday realize the accomplishment of her mom. The world wit-nessed a thrilling, tear-jerking finish. New passions were certainly kindled; race numbers in the sport of triathlon should be up next year as Americans have seen what it's all about.

Women have been participating in the Olympics for a hundred years, starting with the event in 1900 in Paris when nineteen women were there. Every year the number of female competitors has grown; participation in these games was 39% female. We watched well-muscled girls and women exhibit determination, skill, focus and strategy in the summer games of 2000.

They claimed to be a team of gymnasts, but the sprites who hurled and twisted themselves about on the balance beam, the uneven bars, and the floor must constantly squelch a natural tendency of self preservation inherent in every individual's nature. Their guts and solidity pleased and awed us, in spite of falls and fewer medals than wished. We found it ridiculous and sickening to see overweight coach Bella Karolyi react with exasperation when the USA team did not finish as high as he wanted.

But we listened with respect as we heard the story of diver Laura Wilkinson's determination. She had broken her foot in dryland training just months before the games; knowing that the necessary surgery would prevent her from participating, she opted to endure the pain and disfigurement and postpone the operation until the fall of the year. Hobbling up the dozens of steps to the diving platform in a special boot before tossing it to the deck, along with caution, she smiled and plunged from the 10-meter platform into the liquid abyss below. How does it feel to point the toes of a broken foot? Laura did it all right and proceeded to edge out the graceful pair of petite, charming Chinese divers who had dominated the event and claim a gold medal for herself.

Marion Jones had vowed as a little girl of eight that she would be a track star; we were believers when she flashed her golden smile and sprinted to a gold medal in her silver shoes. The strong, beautiful track diva appeared immune to the scandal surrounding her husband and mentor, shot-putter C.J. Hunter, who had tested positive for steroid use; her eyes were trained on five gold medals. Though she came up a bit shy when her long jump, much longer than appeared necessary to win, produced a red flag, a foul, we respected her style and concentration through the controversy. She had class as well as incredible talent.

Though I couldn't get into the funky beach-volleyball mentality, our basketball, softball, water polo, and soccer teams and our swimmers gave us a taste of bravado and nail-biting excitement. Time stood still as girls fought for loose balls and tried to score goals. The world didn't see any more sports bras in the final soccer game for the gold medal, but the point was made that girls can "just do it." It was so cool to know that we had witnessed the first ever women to compete in Olympic weight lifting, pole vault, and hammer throw events.

In spite of these inspiring accomplishments by individuals and teams, the media continued to under-report the female competitors, writing more stories and showing more photographs of males and their sports. Sports Illustrated published its "special Olympic commemorative issue" with twenty-two pages of photographs in 3D, a result of much training with shutter speeds and focal lengths; each magazine contained a pair of complimentary 3D glasses. The effects were quite nice, but it was disappointing to see that there were almost four times the number of these special pictures of males as of females. We need to advocate to increase equity and decrease gender bias both in quality and quantity of sports coverage. No one questions the power of the media and its influence in determining what is important and valuable to us. I watched the Miss America pageant when I was a little girl and wanted to sing, model my swimsuit, and parade down the ramp to the crooning of Bert Parks' "Here she comes...." The seeds of interest were sown in the minds of little girls watching the summer games; the dreams must be encouraged to take hold and grow. And yes, women of all ages can pursue bodies which are strong and healthy - so much more than a sex object!

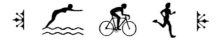

October 2000

*"A man should never be ashamed to own he has been in the
wrong, which is but saying in other words that he is wiser today
than he was yesterday."*

Pope

I was more thorough in sending the itineraries for
our trip to Calais, France, to the three boys, even though
we would be gone only nine days for the International
Triathlon Union (ITU) World Championship Duathlon.
Will was well settled in as a college freshman at Western
Washington University in view of snow-capped Mt.
Baker whose peaks must have been beckoning him to
come ride his snowboard; he worked on his rehabilita-
tion all summer, swimming, working out with weights,
and then riding a bike.

In our last conversation with Keith before we left, he
informed us that he had seen two bobcats while hiking
the day before and was hopeful that he would see some
bears in the Shenandoah (another inspiration of nocturnal demons for me). The bridge on his lower front
teeth had come unglued while he was chewing on a
frozen Power Bar, and he had sampled "the best moon-
shine in the county." I sent another "mail drop" of trail
mix and some maps, labeled "Hold for Thru Hiker," to a
small town post office where he intended to stop in a few
days. A conversation with a friend said that since his
son completed the AT hike three years ago, "There has
been NOTHING he CAN'T do."

A knock on the door. "Bonjour, Madame, Monsieur." I

113

wanted to relish a few more minutes in the crisp, white sheets so thick with starch. Early morning dawned with cool ocean breezes off the English Channel wafting the curtains of our open window; French music was playing softly on our radio when the cafe' au lait and croissants were delivered to the room. We had joined about 100 others on the American duathlon team in Dallas the previous day and flown together to Brussels where we collected our bikes and bags and climbed on a bus for the three hour drive to Calais. Lots of snoring, bobbing heads, and the random alarms of sports watches form my only recollections of the drive, after getting very little sleep on the overseas flight.

The coastal town was alive with excitement over being selected as the venue for this event. Posters decorated street corners with images of cyclists and runners superimposed upon one another. Every traffic circle had been planted with flowers in a myriad of designs, the most memorable being a huge peacock of amazing colors, a few feet away from Rodin's Men of Calais in front of the Town Hall. More than 1,000 competitors and 15,000 spectators were expected.

Many of us were staying in a small village on the outskirts of town, about fifteen minutes from the hotel serving as the headquarters for the American team, adding some difficulty to logistics in accessing the bike mechanic, team messages, and the sports massage, so we had rented a car. Lauren, the only other competitor from Nashville, was staying at our hotel with her mother Sheila. Our first mission, after picking up a baguette, some cheese, and a chocolate pastry, was to drive the bike course, which was reputedly quite hilly and apt to be windy.

There was already a long string of cyclists testing these rumors. After passing three riders stranded by the road with flat tires, I knew that there would be a third hazard, i.e. rocky, rough roads. Poor Steve flagged us down and asked, "I have no more spares - can you possibly fit me and my bike in and give me a ride to my hotel?" Our little Renault, fairly full with the four of us, somehow accommodated Steve and his bicycle, once both wheels were removed. "I feel like hanging these tires over the cross," he added as we topped a hill with yet another lovely white crucifix standing guard. He reminded us of this omen on the bus two days after the race, as he nursed a broken clavicle, the result of sliding out on the last "round-about" of the bike course.

Once Lauren and I had assembled our bikes (I have finally gotten adept at this mechanical part) and pumped our tires, we rode the three miles down to where the bike loop came out from town. As we casually rode, we passed a group of boys walking beside the narrow road. Trying to be friendly, I nodded "bonjour" as one boy smiled and then kicked a coke can directly at our front tires. Lauren and I were able to dodge the can; I don't think he meant any harm, but we were reminded to be vigilant.

On the course, there was one hill over a mile long, leaving me breathless. As we reached the top, a spectacular vista of the white cliffs of Dover beyond the lovely rolling farms and over the sea below caught my attention; then I was instantly negotiating dramatic switchbacks with my hands gripping the brakes. We caught a group of about a dozen French junior cyclists, outfitted in their baby blue uniforms. We tried to communicate in a mixture of English and French. They were interested in my pretty nineteen-year-old companion, and egos emerged; cyclists are notorious for this.

That day I enjoyed my surroundings and the quirks

of a different culture. It would be all business on Saturday when the scenery would be a blur. It had gradually dawned on me that the bike course was shorter than I had thought, only forty kilometers, rather than sixty (twenty-five miles, as opposed to thirty-six); this was a relief when I saw how hard the course would be.

Intending to stay off my feet as much as possible, we planned a day trip two days before the race to see the beaches of Normandy. It was a long drive, and the World War II memorial in Caen didn't get nearly the attention it deserved. But a wonderful lunch in a renovated thirteenth-century farmhouse, finished off with a body- and soul-warming glass of Calvados, and a walk on the beach littered with remains of D-Day landing relics made it worthwhile. We collected a shell as a memento for my father, who had many contemporaries involved in the European theater. This area with its apple trees and lovely cultivated fields of potatoes speaks little today of those awful, bloody days in the 1940s; it would provide a wonderful area for a bicycle trip in the future. We had a fast drive back to Calais so that Johnny could hold the clinic for any athletes needing medical attention and I could get a leg massage.

David is the massage therapist who goes to most of the world championship races. I had enjoyed his help in Perth and was happy that he was in Calais. He gives a deep sports massage; I wanted my legs to be well primed. Because I had signed up late for the event, my name was not on the age-group list, but our team manager Tim assured me that he would handle the necessary details of my registration. There were reports of a strong woman from the Netherlands in my age group.

The day before the race was busy, as usual. We walked to Town Hall to collect race packets, attend the obligatory instructional meetings where rules were explained in French and English, and take the team picture. There was more confusion and less organization than I had found in the Perth race. The running piece of the race was highlighted on a city map and explained to us by Tim. Competitors were not allowed to practice on the course because it was in downtown and there was too much automobile traffic. The race began with two laps of a 5K (3.1 mile) loop, each composed of three spurs off of the main road, running counterclockwise; after the bike ride there was a final 5k run, clockwise. Tim promised, "It's tabletop flat."

The cool weather had turned even cooler, with heavy clouds threatening and rain in the forecast; we were busy converting temperature in degrees from centigrade to Fahrenheit. Discussion centered around what to wear for the race (everything from the skimpy team swimsuit to shorts and the team singlet to tights and gloves ....) We were trying to remember to drink plenty of fluids even though the weather hardly demanded it at the time. Lauren and I wanted to see the first and final five miles of the bike course, with its numerous traffic circles, sharp turns, and narrow roads. So we took the car back to our hotel and pedaled the five miles into town to deposit the bikes in transition.

Transition areas vary a lot from race site to race site; it might be a paved parking lot or a huge grassy field, wet, sandy, or muddy. Competitors often carry a towel and plastic bucket to fill with water for washing their feet off before putting on socks and shoes. Sometimes mats will be laid out to protect competitors from sharp rocks and glass. The Town Hall in center city Calais was the first time I had ever seen a transition area of cobblestones. We would have to run in hard, cleated bike shoes, pushing our bikes, to the point where we would be allowed to mount our bikes.

"Watch out for the glass!" warned a woman in the transition area where I was walking to rack my bike. Lots of broken glass between the stones caught my attention as I found my number on the wooden racks. There were two Frenchmen making their way (at a "pas de probleme" pace) around the huge area with a generator-run vacuum cleaner. A very intense Canadian woman in my age group was hustling around with a toilet brush and a plastic bag in case they never made it to her area. I had visions of a flat tire before I ever left the transition the next morning; I was also sizing her up.

Flags from all participating countries were blowing hard from high wires suspended from a crane above the cobblestones. Our legs were marked with a red pen on the left calf with a number to indicate our age group; women in my age group were marked with #8. We covered our handlebars, computers, and bike seats with plastic bags in case of rain and left the area under the surveillance of numerous muzzled German shepherd dogs.

Johnny and I had a delicious meal of curried vegetables and the wonderful bread you find only in France (I postponed indulging in another delicious French dessert until after the race) in our hotel dining room, where I met Jane. She and her husband had also skipped the parade and "pasta party." I've gone to many of these events and didn't want to be out late. "We're in the same age group - I saw you at the meeting earlier today," she said. Jane looked slim and strong; I hadn't researched the competition very well. The lights were turned out early; unfortunately I didn't sleep well at all. Thank goodness, I had had a good sleep the night before.

Saturday was race day. It was hard to tell in the dark

of dawn how the weather would develop; it wasn't raining, but the morning was quite cool. I decided to wear shorts and the American team singlet to start the run and then to pull on a long sleeved shirt before the bike part of the race. The women started first; three age groups were collected together, so I was grouped with all women over forty. We moved from one "holding area" to another. As we waited, I was able to look around and see the numbers on calves, although a few of the women were wearing tights, hiding their numbers. I lined up in the third row; the only #8 I saw ahead of me was the Canadian woman of glass-cleaning repute.

The start was fast, and I maintained the pace, feeling it was definitely faster than a seven-minute-per-mile pace. A few slowed down, not being able to continue like that. No one passed me. As I completed the first loop, I was surprised to see a sub-20-minute reading on my watch! I was running like that's all I had to do that day - no bike ride, no second 5k run. I continued to run hard and was very aware of who was ahead of me and behind me as I rounded barricades on each spur of the run. I was first of the ten American women and knew of only the Canadian woman ahead (maybe the woman from the Netherlands was wearing tights, covering up her number). As I completed the 10k run in forty minutes, I was thrilled that this was a personal record (PR) for me for a 10k run (I was told later that the course was "short"; it's unbelievable that the measurement is not accurate at a world championship race).

To Johnny's and Sheila's cheers, I quickly got into cycling gear and, looking around and noticing many women in singlets, made a snap decision to leave the long-sleeved shirt behind; that was a mistake. I was well warmed up from the run, but the wind was blowing cold, and the skies were overcast. The weather robbed my body heat; I never felt the goose bumps indicative of hypothermia, but I do think the cool wind sapped some of my power. The bike ride was hard. I passed a few women in younger age groups and was passed by one German woman with a #8, but that was all.

"You're in fourth place, two minutes back, hurry!" Johnny yelled as I rode into transition.

"Go girl," added Sheila. My change to running shoes was quick, and I grabbed a package of chocolate "Gu" for mental support as much as anything. I knew I would have to catch the German if there would be any hope of a medal; but I had a faster run than she did in the 10k, so that would be possible.

Team manager Tim was positioned at the center of the course where he could cheer as we came from each of the spurs on the course. There were four Americans running together near me; they were in the 40-44 and 45-50 age groups. "Put it into the next gear, support each other, you're close!" yelled Tim with only a hundred yards to go. I picked up my pace, gaining on the German, but couldn't change my position more than about 30 seconds.

I crossed the finish line. After a few minutes in the food tent, the results were posted, and I was listed in seventh place. I couldn't imagine where those other women had been! It was starting to rain. The men were out on the course. Lauren had started in a wave ten minutes before me; she had placed second in her field (two seconds behind me in overall time) and would get a silver medal. It's so cool to think that I can compete with a nineteen year old athlete!

My effort had been hard: my legs were tight, and my right arch hurt. I soaked in a hot bath and headed over for David's help. The muscles felt like loaves of thick bread, with lots of whole wheat and whole grains making them heavy. He rubbed them with oil until they were warm, kneaded and stretched them, as I told him about my race. He knows most of the American athletes and told me about our leading male in the 60-64 age group. He knew of one Frenchman ahead of him in the race; when results were posted, there were four others! We had a wonderful post-race dinner, including a French wine and a sinful sundae with warm French chocolate and liqueur over the ice cream.

At breakfast the following morning, Jane's husband Jim approached me. "You had a wonderful race, but I think maybe you were cheated out of a medal." He went on to say that he had been watching every phase of the race very closely, Jane being a few minutes behind me and in my age group. He seemed fairly certain of the competition from other countries.

Johnny and Sheila added to the uncertainty, "We told you there was the Canadian woman and the woman from the Netherlands." Of course, I knew also of the woman from Germany who had passed me on the bike. I called Tim to tell him about this. He felt that maybe some people had been listed in the wrong age groups; he promised to look into it.

"You don't think anyone at this level would cheat, do you?" asked Johnny. Thoughts drifted back to the infamous Rosie Ruiz, who had short-circuited the Boston Marathon course years ago, placing first woman. She was later de-throned. Today, with computerized timing chips, cheating is difficult. I started thinking about the out-and-back spurs of the run course. There were breaks in the barricade all along the road, with very few race officials and no timing checks at the turnarounds. I didn't see anyone cut the course, but it certainly would have been possible.

The junior elites and pros were competing on Sunday; it was rainy, but Johnny had to be at the race to provide medical coverage and we wanted to cheer for the six Americans in the event. We ran into Tim, who said that he had questioned race officials about some of the results. They were offended by his inquiry, saying, "Results were all done by computer chips." Tim told me, "This is Europe. Check the splits on the internet."

That night we went to the hospital to check on one American who had crashed in the rain on the bike course, sustaining a shoulder separation and fracture. He had already had surgery, but he and his wife wanted to ask Johnny some questions.

We extended our trip with a two-day stay in Brussels before flying home. What we found was a city of weird, wild, and wonderful sculpture on every street corner, splashed by the spray of fountains. We studied for hours the works of famous painters in the Museum of Ancient and Modern Art. There was fabulous shopping and delicious food, eaten to the serenade of opportunistic musicians setting up shop on the sidewalks. Johnny was able to see the beautiful gardens of the city on early morning runs, but my legs were still too sore to join him.

As we flew westward home, there was time for reflection, experiencing an endless day over the ocean and in the clouds. I felt a bit like I did a month ago, when I was trying to decide on a dress for the wedding of a good friend. I had a closet full of clothes, but nothing to wear. I had improved my placing in these international events, but I hadn't qualified for the Hawaiian Ironman Triathlon or gotten a medal. The World Championship Duathlon would be on the Mediterranean coast of Italy next fall and the triathlon in Cancun the following spring. I would "age up." I felt a new goal hatching. Of course before either of those races, we had to get ready for the ocean swim in St. Croix in two weeks!

My reverie was broken when we collected our bags in Dallas to clear customs and check them to Nashville. The three suitcases were there, but the bike box was missing. "You'll have to report it at your final destination," said the attendant. Johnny assured me that he had seen the man take the big blue box away with its tag securely attached when we checked in at the Brussels airport.

"You don't think it could be related to the CO2 cartridges, do you?" I asked him. We didn't think so. After the experience in Fiji where the cartridges had been confiscated from my carry-on bag, and the difficulty of finding the item in Perth and in Hawaii, I had decided to pack the small two-inch cylinders in the box with the bike. There had been no problems on the flight home from Hawaii or the flight to Brussels.

I pulled out the four baggage claim stubs and handed them to the woman on duty in the airline missing-baggage office in Nashville. She studied her computer monitor, before looking up. "They kept your bike box in Brussels because you had CO2 cartridges in there," she lectured. "It's illegal and punishable by law to carry any compressed gases. You know they can fine you $10,000;" her voice became louder and her tone more harsh with each word. I didn't say much, but I felt guilty; I'm sure she saw it on my face, and it fed her diatribe.

Johnny pushed open the swinging glass door to enter the office and, catching the gist of her words, joined the conversation in an obligatory defense of his wife. "Where is it written that you can't carry any of these small cartridges?" he demanded.

"Right here," she continued, pointing to the ticket

jacket (and a picture), "and at every ticket counter." Unfinished, her words seemed to gain gravity as she pecked on her computer, "They are even more strict in Europe, and you can expect it in this country. You don't want to get in bad with the FAA (Federal Aviation Authority)!"

At this point I could feel Johnny's position weaken. "It's not my bike!" He backed off a few steps. I wouldn't have been surprised to hear him say, "I really don't know this woman." We were told that the bike would probably be on a flight later that night. Meanwhile, I felt really stupid. Not only had I not learned anything from the experience in Fiji, but I had assured Lauren that it would be fine for her to pack her cartridges with her bike for the flight home.

For the next three days I called frequently about the bike; each time I was told that it would probably be coming later in the day. I began to suspect that they had used the cartridges as an excuse to confiscate the bike and that I'd never see it again. I called Lauren. Thank goodness, her trip had been uneventful; she had wrapped the cartridges up in socks and packed them in her suitcase.

I did get the bike back. The locks had been cut off the case and the cartridges removed, but everything else was accounted for. I never heard a word from the FAA. I once heard someone say that "good judgment" comes from experience, and that experience is the result of bad judgment. Contrary to this popular opinion, many psychologists believe that wisdom is not acquired over the course of a lifetime, but that some people are blessed with more innate wisdom than others. I agree with this; I think I missed that gene. I am sure my three sons would have had something to say about learning from your mistakes!

We had spoken with sons Johnny and Will while we were in France, but hadn't communicated with Keith in two or three weeks. When people heard what Keith was doing, some would say, "He's carrying a cell phone, isn't he?" Without being rude, I informed them that there was no electricity on the trail, no way to recharge a battery for a cell phone. Of course, that was beside the point; he was in the wilderness, trying to escape such trappings of civilization. We had to wait for his move for communicating.

When his call finally came, we talked for a long time. He had seen four wild ponies in the Shenandoah, had finally found someone to resole his boots, and had eaten the traditional obligatory half gallon of ice cream at the midway point "Half-Gallon Challenge." While having lunch with "Easy Rider" at a shelter, they had met the resident rattlesnake. Another hiker (described as "weird") had grabbed Keith's walking stick and used it along with his own to hoist the snake up and threw it away, following up with a death whack. "He's too accustomed to hikers," was the reasoning for the kill.

Keith spoke of the "trail angels." During his journey, many people had gone out of their way with small and large acts of kindness. There was the man who volunteered to drive him twenty-plus miles up the highway (and back to the trail) to the church where Keith's great-great-great grandparents are buried. Churches offered free lodging, laundry facilities and meals for "thru-hikers." The simple gesture of supplying toilet paper to outhouses was a blessing. There was the couple who drove his package to a point further along the trail to deliver it personally because the post office had been closed for a holiday when he hiked through town. I sensed that my son's words were spoken to me with a smile on his lips, the experience enriching his soul. The journey had become a metaphor of life, with its ups and downs, some days silky smooth and others as rough as a pineapple.

At this point we had all realized that he would not be finishing the walk until December. "Since you won't be home for Thanksgiving, we will bring Thanksgiving to you."

"That sounds great!" said "Old man Sam."

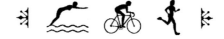

November 2000

"Remote for detachment,
narrow for chosen company,
winding for leisure,
lonely for contemplation,
the Trail
leads not merely north and south,
but upward to the body, mind, and soul of man."

Myron Avery
The Appalachian Trail
Conference

October, the month of the World Championship Hawaiian Ironman Triathlon, had come and gone. We received word that Ray had a hard time. He had swallowed a lot of salt water during the swim which made him sick, and he had became dehydrated as a result. Mechanical problems with his bike brought additional insult. He had to quit; this was his first DNF (Did Not Finish). His analysis was "four for me, one for Kona." I heard that he doesn't plan to go back. On the other hand, Sandi from Vancouver (who beat me at the Keahou-Kona race in May) had a good day, finishing first in our age group of about thirty competitors; the woman from Oregon who had beaten me the year before in Buffalo Springs, Texas, placed second. Obviously, I kept picking qualifying races with the toughest competition!

Training for the swim in St. Croix got serious. Carol had us doing two miles at each session on Monday, Wednesday, and Friday mornings. She became a strict task-master, but she remained our friend and our inspiration. Having discovered that she carries the BRCA1 gene mutation and knowing that her twin brother died of colon cancer at a young age and that her mother was in the final stages of ovarian and breast cancer, she had elected to have a prophylactic total mastectomy as soon as we returned from the trip to St. Croix, a reconstruction the following spring, and a oophyrectomy (removal of the ovaries) the following summer.

Johnny couldn't swim with the group due to his work. His forearm was bothering him ("tennis elbow") because he hadn't been swimming regularly for months, and he wasn't used to these workouts. Together we gave him a cortisone shot in his elbow! It would be a five mile swim. Some planned to do the whole distance, and the rest of us would form three-person teams, each individual doing a 1.7 mile leg. I kept up my running and biking in the beautiful, warm autumn days. Not feeling pressured to ride hard, we sought out roads I'd never ridden and took in a glorious fall.

Of the fifteen going to St. Croix from Nashville, at least half had never done any open-water swimming and were nervous about the tides, the currents, salt water, and the sea life (especially sharks). We had lots of reassuring conversations and a slide show highlighting what creatures to look for underwater. One of the TV stations came out to the pool, filmed us training, and interviewed several of us. The three-minute segment came on at 11:30 pm, after an hour's discussion of professional football and after most people were in bed.

I called Lois a few days before our trip. Lois had been battling breast cancer. Diagnosed ten years before, she had undergone a mastectomy and chemotherapy and believed she had achieved a cure. But last spring the beast had reared its ugly head again; her doctors told her she had maybe six months to live. She sat up one night out of her sleep and knew that she needed to go to Africa, the origin of life as we know it. We worried that she was going there to die. Wrong! She was going there to live, which we learned when we went to her house to see the pictures of the animals and lands of the safari she and Wayne photographed. Since then they have been to Alaska and the Smoky mountains. Ten days in Florida was next on their agenda. "The cancer is reduced by three-fourths," she shared. "I have quality of life. I'm running two miles a day. Friends ask me why I'm doing it. I tell them it makes me feel good."

Lois knew that we had gone to the South Pacific in the spring, and I shared with her that we had just returned from France a few weeks before. "I'm embarrassed to tell people that we leave for St. Croix in two days," I added. "People must wonder how we can afford it."

"Whatever it takes, do these things. You never know what tomorrow will bring!" Her words were spoken from experience and salved my conscience.

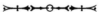

The fifth annual St. Croix Reef Swim took place from Buck Island, an uninhabited island more than a mile and a half off the north shore of the main island, to the Buccaneer Hotel, with 180 swimmers participating. There were ten relay teams, a fin division, and the rest were solo swimmers. Competitors came from Puerto Rico, Belgium, France, Mexico, Canada, Germany, and the United States, as well as the Virgin Islands. The youngest swimmer was just ten years old, and several were in their 70's.

Our group from Nashville arrived during the three

days prior to the event. We went out to Buck Island, a white sand beach, voted one of the most pristine by National Geographic, for a morning of snorkeling to see the starting location before race day. We paddled on the water's surface around "the guided path" of an underwater park, spotting a huge green moray eel hiding in a coral hole, a large lobster, and lots of colorful fish. The humor of the day evolved as we tried repeatedly to stage a photo with our underwater camera. Arms and legs splashed in all directions as we attempted to have everyone get a breath and go under and "smile," forming a nice "group shot."

Johnny and I went scuba diving one morning, enjoying underwater life quite different from what we had seen in Fiji. There were sea fans, forests of coral with branches bending in the current, hundreds of tropical fish, some in schools, others darting alone, bearing names like parrot, jewel and angel. Brilliant blues, yellows, and greens, they did their own dance; the little six-inch damsel fish actually attempted to pick a fight with me. The divemaster and captain of the boat predicted that there would be no sharks to worry about for the Sunday swim, but maybe some turtles, rays, and jellyfish to entertain us.

We took advantage of off-season golf rates and the under-used course and played nine holes; at least we hacked away at nine holes. I hit some occasional good shots and lots of bad ones, not bothering to tally my score. Liz is a talented golfer and gave us some tips; Richard inaugurated a brand new set of clubs, amusing us with a couple of shots when he skipped a ball four or five times across a pond, sending the swimming cattle egrets either diving under the water or into the air in panicked flight. Johnny sent dozens of frigate birds flying, when he hit their nesting tree, not once, but twice, losing both balls in the hazard below. The hilly course treated us to gently blowing trade winds and spectacular views.

St. Croix, a little island of only eighty four square miles, has an interesting history. It is proud to have been the landing site of Christopher Columbus in 1493. Seven flags fly over its government buildings, representing the countries and privateers under which it has suffered and prospered through the years. A lilting version of English, defined linguistically as Creole and commonly called Calypso, is spoken throughout the West Indies with variations from one island to another. Many Americans live on the island, taking advantage of tax cuts and the benefits of a laid-back, stress-free lifestyle. We enjoyed conversations with local inhabitants and were invited for cocktails at a hillside home of some Nashvillians with business on the island.

We did some shopping in the boutiques and listened to steel pan bands. A visit to the "Parrot" music shop involved conversing with locals concerning their favorite reggae and purchasing several CD's for the boys and ourselves. We indulged in delicious food. Origins of the island cuisine are from African and West Indian island traditions; many names sounded strange (kallaloo, goat water and maubi), and the locally-made hot sauces were served without warning, sending me for water after I added a healthy spoonful to my omelette. Fresh grilled fish and lobster bisque were savored, along with island fruits and pastries. There were even opportunities for "cheeseburgers in Paradise"! The mellow, smooth rum made on the island was consumed in drinks for which there was no recipe; any kind of fruit juice would suffice, as long as there was plenty of ice and a cherry. We walked over yellow bricks carted from Dutch ships and under gracefully-arched, sheltered sidewalks protecting us from the hot sun or a momentary shower.

All in all the tropical days and nights were splendid. We had come for the experience; not being highly competitive meant we didn't suffer from the usual pre-race jitters and could relax more. Which brings up a topic which causes us all to balk and be embarrassed - love life and sex after menopause (and/or hysterectomy). We are sexual beings from day one, and this does not change as we age, whether we are single or with a spouse or partner. Decreased vaginal lubrication and the thinning of the vaginal walls from reduced estrogen levels may cause penetration to be uncomfortable, and less blood flow to the genital area makes orgasms seem less intense. Water-based lubricants, such as Astroglide which was inspired by the lube NASA used for the O-rings on space shuttles, are helpful and easily washed out of bed sheets. The pleasure of oral sex may be rediscovered, and "dildos" (they make people nervous but they've been around in one form or another since the beginning of civilization) can help keep vaginas toned, as can masturbation (it does not cause blindness or insanity and was declared in 1972 by the American Medical Association to be a normal sexual activity). The kids being out of the house, the freedom from the fear of getting pregnant, or a long-awaited retirement provide a good time to work on communication with our partner and getting over our hangups. Here again, "use it or lose it" - and don't underestimate the psychological power of memory and habit. Somehow most women know intuitively that having a "sex life" is desirable, providing not only the warmth and tenderness of touch, but vitality and a connection to others.

My only problem was with itching from the bites on my ankles and toes. I had learned that there were mosquitoes, sugar-ants, and no-see-ums on St. Croix. Some of us are more attractive to these pests than others, a function of body chemistry and temperature. Studies have shown that in a group of people exposed, about one-third will be bitten many times, one-third will be untouched, and the rest will receive a bite or two. I must belong to that first population. I never saw what bit me, but the result was horrible. I found some relief from aloe and "Tea Tree Spirit," an "all natural antiseptic" product from Australia, but the salt water in the ocean was the best treatment.

On the afternoon before the race we picked up our race packets and attended the required meeting. Pre-race meetings are all different! There we were with a red sunset at our backs, a breeze blowing the palm trees and waves lapping the Caribbean beach two hundred feet below the open-air hotel terrace. The race director grew sentimental, wiping his eyes, when he introduced special people in the audience, including Mr. O'Brien, who won the gold medal for the shot put in the Olympics in 1952 and 1956, the bronze four years later, and placed fourth the following year. Then the speaker turned humorous in his instructions, making jokes, and everyone laughed. I thought he was kidding when he mentioned a weather report of six foot ocean swells; he didn't laugh.

There had been some discussion concerning who should do each leg of our relay. The first leg, considered the hardest, would be from Buck Island over to the main island, the current pushing from east to west, actually a little longer than the other two legs at 1.8 miles. The final two legs would parallel the coast and were predicted to have the benefit of a prevailing current. Carol felt that I should do the first leg. I had the benefit of more training, as well as experience. Johnny felt, on the other hand, that because I am nearsighted and do have trouble with sighting distances that maybe he should do the first leg. It was decided that I would take the boat out for the start, Judy would do the middle leg, and Johnny would do the final one.

We trundled out into the star-studded dark on race morning. Our arms were marked, and we were loaded on boats for the ride over to the island or to the boat where we would be waiting for our teammate. The time on the boat ride was spent lathering up with sunscreen, drinking water and sports drinks, and discussing strategy. Lyndell, Katherine, Holli, and I discussed swimming along together. There were supposedly three large boats which we should keep to our right and a final large sailboat marking the point where we would tag our next swimmer. One bronzed gentleman who bore a countenance of experience was sipping a beer! He was obviously there for a good time.

The start was initiated with the blowing of a conch shell. As a helicopter flew overhead, I swam right over a scuba diver filming from below the water. There were dozens of kayakers there in case of trouble. In the swarm of swimmers I lost sight of Lyndell, Katherine, and Holli and proceeded on my own. We had been advised to sight on the pink condominiums on the far shore, allowing the current to push us in the direction of the sailboat indicating the turn. Going straight for the turn boat might result in being washed to the right of these boats. I swam steadily, enjoying sights of hundreds of five-pointed starfish, almost making me question which way was up, and a stingray on the ocean floor. The swells were huge; it was impossible to see the boats on my right when I lifted my head to sight, but I felt comfortable. There were other swimmers and a kayak near me. I realized that I had swum too close to shore when I started seeing lots of sea urchins in the coral just a few feet below in shallow water.

I looked at my watch; I'd been swimming for an hour. "Where's the sailboat?" I yelled at one of the other swimmers near me.

"I was following you; I thought you knew," she responded.

"Where's the boat?" I yelled at the kayaker. He pointed downshore about a half mile. In a triathlon a kayaker would have volunteered the information and yelled at a swimmer if you were going off course.

After fifteen more minutes of serious swimming, I reached the sailboat and tagged Judy who had a worried look on her face. "What happened to you?" I gave her a quick explanation of "getting off course," and she took off. Lyndell and Katherine had reached the boat several minutes before me. Holli had had the same trouble I did, but we had not even seen each other in that huge expanse of water. Stories were shared as reggae played from the boat's sound system. There were reports of pulling one harried woman out. Another woman in the fin division had climbed on a kayak when she realized she was literally "in over her head." We threw water bottles to the five-mile swimmers as they passed the boat. Katherine, the most fearful of ocean creatures, had seen a shark! Her story was later corroborated by the overall winner who had also seen it.

We sailed back to the dock to see the finishers swim in to the beach. Our coach Carol was third overall female in the five-mile swim! The three top relay teams were youngsters from the islands. We had finished sixth out of ten teams. I didn't feel bad about that, but Johnny was disgruntled. He said that he was worried that I had trouble in the ocean when Judy was slow in coming to tag him. And he felt that he would have been able to swim a straighter course. Personally, I believe he was suffering from a male-gender-specific macho attitude.

They say that wallpapering is the leading cause of divorce; we had experience with that activity about twenty-five years before. Our solution was to finish papering half of the ceiling and paint the rest. A few years earlier we had experienced some marital strife when we were paddling a two-person canoe on the rapids of the Hiawassee River, where we had joined a weekend course on whitewater technique. Steering from the stern, Johnny was yelling "paddle harder on the right, now the left, no the right...!" I was yelling at him to paddle straight! He succeeded in wedging us upright on a ledge in the middle of the river, with water raging on both sides. When we finally climbed out of the boat, not speaking to each other, the leader put us in different boats for the rest of the weekend.

We now hire someone else to do the wallpapering, and we paddle single kayaks. Now I have added to that list not being on the same swim relay team! We all know that marriage is not a case of unadulterated happiness, but rather a series of peaks and valleys. We're actually in sympatico most of the time; our roots have grown deeper over our 33 years together. Our marriage, like all, will continue to meet new sets of stresses with each of life's transitions (midlife, empty-nest, elderly and passing of parents, menopause, ...) so our "bank account" needs periodic emotional and physical deposits. I had actually been looking forward to pedaling a tandem bicycle with him! Could be a mistake - but I want to try.

Our flight home was late in the day, allowing a group of us to take a casual ocean kayaking tour on the island (we were put in a canoe together and got along fine).

Andy, an MBA-graduate who moved to the island to escape a stressful job of negotiating arms deals between the U.S. and Israel, and Jennifer, who also works with her boyfriend at the island aquarium, were our guides. They took the group through mangrove swamps and educated us about the flora, the fauna, and the ravages of Hurricane Hugo in 1989. Andy told us that there was not a blade of grass or a tree standing when he went out of his door the morning after the storm pounded the island. We saw the hulls of what were once beautiful boats still stranded lopsided against the shore. The birds had started to return and swamps were recovering their vital role of providing spawning grounds for ocean life and protection of the sand beaches.

As we flew home, an effervescent gentleman from Belgium struck up a conversation (under the guise of an interest in my computer report of "the swim"). He does open water swimming all winter long, breaking the ice when necessary. When we asked if he wears a wetsuit, he sneered, "I use only grease, ... don't cheat." He had done the entire five miles using the breaststroke and complained that the water was "too hot, causing much sweating."

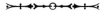

While we were gone, the first Canadian cold front had blown in from the north; the fall leaves of red and gold had turned a dull brown, floating down and crumbling on the ground below the woody skeletons of winter. Summer clothes were washed and put away. We didn't plan late afternoon bike rides anymore; it was too cold and dark. But we continued to swim and run.

Each season gives different gifts to the runner. As we started a park run one fall morning with just the right conditions, we were surprised to see surrounding us throughout the woods the stems of dead wildflowers and grasses wrapped in an ethereal white gauze called hoarfrost. Known by some as "rabbit ice," it forms when moisture or fog becomes a solid and splits the stems, oozing out as frozen white pillows, spongy and soft in our fingers as we slowed to feel it. When the temperature rose a few degrees, our icy paradise vanished; however, the warmer air produced yet another offering from Mother Nature - the acrid sweet odor of fallen persimmons being crushed under our feet in a fermenting forest.

We shared our trip pictures with friends. Little by little we started talking about what we would do next season. Rusty called with registration information about the Vineman Half-Ironman Triathlon in California; it would fill up quickly so we sent in our applications.

To prepare for the Thanksgiving feast with Keith on the Trail I cooked and froze some of the boys' favorite holiday foods: cornbread dressing with pecans and sausage, fudge and pumpkin pies, and green beans. Johnny experimented with smoking a turkey; we sampled it, found it delicious, and froze it.

Keith called two weeks before Thanksgiving to discuss where we might rendezvous. He estimated how long the hike would take him, how we could access the trail by car, and settled on Hot Springs, North Carolina, one of a handful of towns where the trail actually comes right through town. I located a perfect rental unit with a kitchen in the small town; it was called "The Short Porch." He gave me a list of things to bring when we came instead of mailing the items. The list included his down jacket which he had sent back during the warm summer months and his gaiters to keep water and snow out of his boots. Suddenly the weather got bitterly cold, dropping down into the low twenties in Nashville, which meant it was probably much colder in the mountains. I tried not to think about it, but I was worried about him, imaging a son shivering with frostbite.

A call came two days before our scheduled meeting. The temperature had gotten down to twelve degrees, and it had been snowing but Keith assured us that he was fine. He told us of hiking solo under a full moon while it was snowing in a pristine spruce forest. He had taken a day off to warm up and spend time with some old high school friends. This had put him behind schedule; he had forty miles to cover in the next two days. "It's not a problem," he assured us. "I'll be there. Is it OK if a few of my friends from the Trail join us for our meal?"

"How many is 'a few'?" Asked Johnny.

"Oh, at least ten, no more than fifteen. And I have been dreaming of a pecan pie; would it be too much trouble for you to make one? By the way, these folks can eat a lot."

About four hundred individuals hike the trail from south to north each year, but less than a hundred do the trip from north to south. So it was about twenty percent of the entire year's ledger of south-bound hikers who would be coming to our Thanksgiving feast. Will flew home from school the night before Thanksgiving, Johnny smoked another turkey, and I cooked a ham, sweet potatoes, and a pecan pie.

Hot Springs is a small town nestled in a circle of the southern Appalachian Mountains on the banks of the French Broad River, about thirty-three miles northwest of Asheville, where the locals claim that "the Goddess of Nature waved her Magic Wand." In the 1700's, the whistle stop was named Warm Springs, emphasizing its mineral waters, rather than its location along the railroad. Numerous hotels were built on the scenic river banks, to draw folks to the area, only to burn to the ground one by one. The town fathers changed the name to Hot Springs (they turned up the thermostat to pull in more tourists). People came on horseback from far and wide to the medicinal mecca. German prisoners of war were housed there in 1917. In place of the hotel there's now a campground. The "metropolis" caters to paddlers, as well as hikers, with a well-equipped outdoor gear store, a small grocery, a pub, a diner, a laundromat, an ATM, a post office, and a hikers' hostel.

We arrived in town early Thursday afternoon, unpacked our food, putting some of it in the oven on low heat, and laced up our hiking boots. A sign was posted at the hostel, according to Keith's instructions, inviting his friends to come for dinner "with Sam's parents at 6:30 or 7:00 pm at 'The Short Porch.'" There was some uncertainty on our part; what if we started hiking and never saw him? We devised a plan to carry paper, a pen, and yellow ribbon. After an hour, if we didn't meet up, we would write a note telling him we had gone to prepare dinner and tie the message with a ribbon to a tree.

As we headed out onto the road to look for the white blazes guiding us to the Trail, a hiker strolled into town. Long hair held in check by a bandana, a beard, hiking poles, and a large backpack with sandals and water bottles dangling from a carabiner - all were a dead giveaway that he was one our son's cohorts.

"Do you know 'Sam'?" I asked.

"Oh, yes, he's my friend." He smiled as he extended his hand. "We spent last night at the same shelter, but I left this morning before he was up."

We learned that this fellow's name was "Still Searching." We told him that we hoped to see him later and moved toward the trail. That was good news.... Keith couldn't be far behind! The trail, well-worn and marked, ambled along the banks of the river before it started climbing. We followed the switchbacks up the mountain for a few miles before meeting another hiker. For a brief second I thought it was my boy ... same coloring to the beard and hair ... five months since I had seen him. But it was another of Keith's friends!

"Do you know 'Sam'?" I quizzed again.

"Oh, are you Sam's family? He told me you were coming. I waited around while I was eating lunch and practicing, but he didn't come. He's probably only about fifteen minutes back." Along with the usual paraphernalia, this hiker had a tuba stuck in the top of his pack, crammed full of clothes! We didn't dilly-dally, but invited "Tuba Man" to our dinner and took off. We moved along quickly and silently; even Uta sensed our attempt to surprise. But down a long stretch, he saw us at just the same second that we saw him, so naturally. A warm smile and long tight hugs.

There were nineteen very smelly bodies, very friendly souls at our Thanksgiving meal. I've never witnessed such caloric capacity; manners were intact but the consumption was enormous. No cloth napkins and freshly-polished silver were at this celebration; it rather reminded me of serving at the shelter for the homeless! We reveled in stories of life on the Trail told well into the night. "Teacup," a sprightly college graduate, was working on her dreadlocks and her future. "Big Man" planned to start a company building custom bicycle frames. "Mo," a special education teacher, and Bill, an accountant, had been traveling the Trail together for five months, solving all kinds of problems, but were still uncertain of marriage. Our sons Will and Keith drifted off to sleep talking about hiking the John Muir Trail and going to Scotland to climb next summer. I asked them how they planned to finance these endeavors.

Keith washed his clothes (I doubt that the dirt will ever really come out) and found a place to check his e-mail the following morning. Then we went to soak in the hot mineral baths. Over the years, grateful testimonials have been offered by visitors, telling of their relief from rheumatism, arthritis, stomach, liver and gallbladder ailments after soaking in and drinking the waters. A worn-out hiker, an injured snowboarder, and their ama-teur-athletic parents went to test the claims. This was actually quite a commercial establishment, with indi-vidual jacuzzi tubs cordoned off in three-sided, seclud-ed wooden fences along the edge of the river. The 100-degree mineral water was piped up to the tubs, and after our prepaid hour of soaking and sipping the waters, the tub was slowly drained out.

"You know, my knee actually feels better," Will chuck-led and smiled. He was bearing witness after partaking of the waters! The screws in his knee still bothered him. He admitted to being sore from his first attempt at skate-boarding since his spring accident. There was little con-versation about when he might strap on his snowboard. After we toweled off and dressed, we left to listen to some bluegrass at the pub.

Keith worked on his boots, waterproofing them again, gluing a loose sole and inserting some screws. He estimated that he would finish his hike in two to three weeks. We discussed driving down to meet him at Springer Mountain in northern Georgia. Several others might need a shuttle into town where they would scatter to different points of civilization.

We drove "Sam" to the edge of town where the trail slips into the woods, marked by 2-inch by 6-inch white blazes painted on the trees. Pictures were snapped as he hoisted up his pack (much heavier with leftover ham, cranberry-nut bread, rolls). Uta followed him happily up through the trees; she would have loved to continue with him for the last 274 miles. That would have been a real possibility except that dogs are not allowed in the Smoky Mountains National Park; fines run $500.

"Call her back," he yelled, "and hey, Dad, how about a few bars from 'Happy Trails.'" (Their father is a closet singer/musician.)

My eyes grew moist as we all chimed in, "Happy trails to you, until we meet again. Happy trails to you, keep smiling until then ...."

Will returned to Washington to finish his term before the Christmas holidays, and we retreated into our "empty nest."

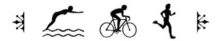

December 2000

⊱┈◈┈◯┈◈┈⊰

"The vehicle is the body, motored by the mind,
fueled by the Spirit"

> Sister Madonna Buder
> Age 70, Catholic nun
> 7-Time Age-group World
> Champion Triathlete

I entered the annual Rudolph-the-Red-Nosed-Reindeer 5k race which precedes the Christmas parade on the first Sunday of December. Cold and damp conditions didn't discourage enthusiastic participation in the costume category; there were jolly Santas, thin and fat, jogging elves, and teams of antlered critters pulling sleighs. My tights and Gortex jacket looked boring, but spectators along the route provided unconditional support. My legs were a little sluggish, from several months of no speed work or races, but I mustered a sub-twenty-two minute time, averaging a little over seven minutes a mile on the hilly course. I won't deny that it hurt; even a short race hurts if you push yourself. Somehow the pain makes great thoughts possible if you don't allow the negative to creep in. I absorbed the sights, the sounds, the smells, and made them a part of my focus. Visiting with friends, collecting a tree ornament for placing first in my age group, and sipping hot chocolate kindled the Christmas spirit.

I started my shopping and cooking for the holidays. My friend Cathy and I spent an afternoon assembling the gingerbread log-houses which has become a tradition for us to launch our seasonal activities. Another friend Allison and her daughter joined in the kneading, cutting, and decorating, creating a kitchen replete with odors of cinnamon and nutmeg, floured aprons, and sticky red sprinkles. A long afternoon of baking provided an opportunity for philosophical musings among chatty girls. "I feel like we're all getting older; I don't think we should even wear shorts anymore," offered Allison.

I was shocked! This came from a very pretty brunette who had been city tennis champ as a teenager. She walks regularly for exercise; granted she is a few pounds heavier now. "Allison, you are dead wrong," I countered. "Please don't assume this mindset. You are very healthy and can feel as fit as you did when you were winning all those tennis matches!"

I knew that I was in the best shape of my life and that other women, even in their years after menopause, have this capability at their fingertips, given the desire and the direction. Years of practice in managing jobs, children, homes, and husbands have made us accountable and responsible. Money spent for a personal trainer (maybe for just a limited time if finances are an issue), a club membership, and a supportive group of friends are building blocks which can foster a new, more active lifestyle.

My mother began to panic about finding gifts for her eight grandchildren and great-grandson and sought help with her shopping. She was worried about her short-term memory loss and spoke to my sister and me about this; she believed that she had perhaps had some "mini strokes." We had been noticing how she repeated herself, telling us the same things over and over again. Ever an energetic optimist, she had nevertheless quit attending her book club, her church circle, and her garden club meetings. Her doctor suggested some psychiatric testing, which we encouraged; but my father, fearing the unknown, didn't want her to proceed with the testing. She also complained of dizziness; her doctor prescribed yet another drug. At this point she was slugging down more than a dozen pills a day, and our father had her "resting" most of the day.

I eventually convinced her to see a psychiatrist under the guise of getting help with her trouble sleeping. A few simple questions and tests dispelled her fears. "I do not think you have had a stroke, and you don't have Alzheimer's. You have what most folks your age have, when it comes to memory - a storage problem. (I was thinking: is it a storage problem I have when I soap my legs in the shower and can't remember if I washed under my arms?) You're not interested in the things you used to enjoy; your life is going backwards."

He prescribed an antidepressant that would also help her sleep and an exercise program. "I want you walking 15 miles a week; I want you to consider a day without exercise as a bad day! It'll help you sleep better without medication since you'll be tired, and improve your circulation, thereby reducing the dizziness, build strength and prevent falls."

Wow, my mother had seen me exercising all those years, reaping so many benefits, and my father was walking a mile in the mall each morning, but neither of us had made it our mission to convince her of the benefits of making exercise a priority. She finally had a plan and a goal, those critical elements to any change in behavior. She started walking in the mall with my father every day.

"I walk faster than Daddy," she said proudly a few days later, not bragging, just matter-of-factly. Within days her mood was elevated; I saw that old glint in her green eyes. She got excited about getting a hot tub and a new kitchen floor. I knew that I needed to convince her of the value of doing some weight-resistance training. With a sedentary lifestyle, her muscle mass had decreased and was making her more and more susceptible to falls.

My father, ever the lawyer at eighty-four, was mesmerized by our never-ending presidential election and concentrated his legal brain on the twenty-four-hour-a-day media coverage. It was the year of butterfly ballots, hanging chads, undercounted, miscounted and recounted votes, as the electoral reptiles couldn't bring Florida into the twenty-first century. While speaking with my mother one morning during the final days of the Gore-Bush standoff, she said, "Your father was so disgruntled this morning. The man who is going to clean our gutters called and woke him out of his dreams. Your dad thought he was being called to Washington to serve as a justice on the Supreme Court deciding the Florida case."

Maybe we should scrap our elections and just let these nine men select our President every four years! My parents continue to provide me with a new perspective on so many issues (in spite of some minor disagreements), and I prayed they would stay in good health for many more years to come.

Late in the night a week later, our oldest son burst into the front door. Startled from the early stages of sleep, we recognized his voice right away. "I can't put up with 'things' in New York any more," announced John. He had driven home. He said he didn't plan to finish the semester in art school, would get a job to make enough money to move back up to work in the city in about a month. He wanted to be free of us, felt he would do better if he were responsible for himself.

Delving gently into these "things" got us nowhere. He claimed that his relationship with his girlfriend was not the reason he had left, that he had missed some classes and that, though his grades weren't great, he hadn't "failed out."

Parents care and worry so much for their children, balancing a fine line between discipline and nurturing. We want them to expand their horizons. How do we communicate to them what degree of verticality, what limits of experimentation, are acceptable? I didn't ask many questions that night, opting to curl up under a blanket in his room and just "be there." I feared that there was something that he was not telling us. He visited friends the next day and stayed out "bowling" until early the next morning. Did I sleep well? I don't think so! I gradually became angry over this situation.

He's an artist, I'm a pragmatist; we've had our battles through the years. So creative, he was born with a style which cannot be taught. At the age of five, when most kids have their lemonade stands, he sat at a card table by the side of the road, cigar box for change, with his drawings and watercolors displayed for sale. As a third grader, his "Machine Gun Man" caught the attention of the featured artist at the school Arts Festival. She wanted it, offering him the chance to pick anything from her studio in exchange. I chose a watercolor of three little boys playing soccer for him. Maybe some day he'll be a famous painter with his own studio, this prize hanging on the wall.

So I said, in essence, "We've paid so much money for you to go to this school; you said you wanted to do this, and you're just blowing us off." We wanted to get our money's worth from his education in some concrete way.

"But I have learned so much this semester whether I

get the credits or not" was his retort. This fell on unsympathetic ears. The decibels in my voice were rising as I continued along my line of reason.

"I would understand it if you told us you were very sick, depressed, or having a big problem. If not, you need to get your butt back up there (I don't usually talk this way) and finish the semester. You'll be halfway toward your degree." By this point, I was screaming, even though I knew from past experience this approach never worked. We offered to buy him a round trip airline ticket. He refused; I fumed. Thank goodness, husband Johnny kept cool, listening rather than vocalizing.

Either my rampage or his late night conversation with his girlfriend made John change his mind. He accepted the offer to fly up to finish the semester. "Don't go if you're just going to find out you've failed everything," I said.

"That's not going to happen," he sounded assured. He left. Meanwhile Will arrived home for Christmas. He felt good about his first college term, was gaining strength in his injured knee and was planning to take some snowboarding gear back out to school for the winter. Though he wouldn't compete, he planned to get back out on the slopes.

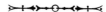

The weather since Thanksgiving had continued to dip to record low temperatures all through the southeast. It was the coldest November and December in over a hundred years. Several fellow AT hikers, with whom Keith had bonded, pooled their resources to share hotel rooms more frequently to keep warm in towns along the trail. A predicted day of pick-up had been made, and then changed; the going was slow when walkers must make fresh tracks in the snow.

It was a frigid, blustery Sunday that greeted the four of us (Johnny, Will, Uta, and me) when we rose early to drive to the north Georgia mountains to collect our son from the Trail. Despite the treacherous driving conditions, we started a trip over icy roads. We had no choice but to go; there was no way to contact him. Our route took us over the Cumberland plateau, a lovely stretch of highway littered with gravel pullouts for runaway trucks and infamous for accidents. The final part of the Appalachian Trail is accessed by seven miles of winding forest service road, that day through snowy woods.

"How's the road ahead?" we asked as we pulled over to let a four-wheel-drive truck pass us on their way out. "There's a tree in the road 'bout a mile before the parking lot," the driver warned. We'd probably have to hike more than we had planned. Another woodsman (actually two good old' boys drinking beer) had cut and moved the tree by the time we got to that point.

We arrived at the parking lot that crosses the Trail one mile from the top of Springer mountain an hour later than the planned rendezvous time. As we braced against the twelve degree temperature and Heaven-only-knows what wind chill factor, we pulled on our jackets, hats, gloves, and boots, grabbed the bottle of celebratory champagne, and looked up to see "Sweat-Box" coming up the Trail. His beard was caked with ice, and he had a "far-off" look in his eyes; he was oblivious to the cold as he made his final walk. "Sam is a few minutes ahead, probably at the top waiting for you."

It was fact; Keith had made it! We hustled up the Trail behind Keith's friend, watching him limp beneath the weight of his pack. His feet must have been so cold; he had done his entire hike in "tennis shoes." We met "Little Debbie" and "the Candyman," two of Keith's good friends who had missed our Thanksgiving feast, coming back down to the parking lot. They would be joining us for the trip back to Nashville, where her father would meet them, driving down from Cincinnati.

Uta found him first; rather, he heard Uta coming. She was wearing her red Christmas collar with jingling bells. Keith was already celebrating with a bottle of cold bubbly champagne, dripping enthusiastically all down his beard, shared with "Teapot," "Wetfoot," and "Gasket." They had taken pictures with their sock-covered hands (they admitted to leaving their now frozen gloves out in the rain two nights before). We all admired the bronze sign marking the start of the long trail and took more pictures before heading down to the car.

We crammed the car with bodies and backpacks, throwing our olfactory senses into overload. The sun shone, melting the snow and making the return drive less difficult; we were entertained for hours by stories of the Trail as the three chronically calorically-depleted hikers munched continuously on snacks. Little Debbie, a petite young woman with a pack every bit as heavy as the largest male's, said she had recently started despising the word "gap" - it meant mountainous terrain had to be covered. They described sharing their shelters in the Smokies with obnoxious mice which would find their way into food bags, having the gall to leave their feces behind! "Gasket" had a record of killing eleven gutsy rodents in two hours to provide his fellow campers in a shelter a more peaceful (and cleaner) night's sleep.

Keith adjusted well to reentering civilization, humbly accepting congratulations from many friends and relatives. He was proud that he had done the whole trail without "slack-packing" any part; in other words, he had not skipped a single mile, and no one had carried his pack ahead for him. He relished showing his six-hundred-odd pictures, explaining them, and putting them into albums. He sent and received e-mail messages from fellow hikers and planned his classes for returning to school in January.

>-!-+>-•-O-•-<+-!-<

My running and swimming training continued, largely unchanged by the seasons. A goal to learn something new is usually energizing, preventing burnout with the routine. I determined to improve my back-stroke and to master the "flip-turn" in the pool. Of the four main swim strokes, the freestyle (the "crawl") is generally the fastest for most people. Training only freestyle, though, can lead to overuse injury - usually in the shoulders - from so much repetition, not to mention boredom. Practicing the other strokes improves one's "feel" for the water; becoming a faster swimmer means learning to propel yourself through the water in different body positions. Open turns can be about as fast as a flip, but the swimmer does lose momentum, and the faster swimmers gained on me with each turn. Mastery of new techniques takes much repetition; I was no exception. I would flip, push off from the wall and come up crooked and gasping for air. After each work-out I left the pool with a stopped-up head and a nasal twang from the repeated chlorinated nose "enemas" of my efforts. But I kept trying, waiting for the light to dawn. I got back to regular workouts with weights; the off-season is a good time to build strength.

Women may eschew time spent in a chlorinated pool and doing activities outside which cause sweat to "mess up" their hair; likewise, they may believe that the cold wind and sun are too harsh and drying for the skin. I have found that showering immediately after any kind of workout and shampooing with a gentle product keeps my hair from being brittle and damaged. Lots of women athletes let their hair grow long enough to do a "pony-tail," but I prefer a short haircut which can be blown dry in a few minutes. Hydration is important for the hair and skin, even in the winter, when moisture is lost through exhalation. Sweat, which is basically salt, is actually good for the scalp! A conditioner and plenty of moisturizing lotion will keep the hair and skin healthy and shiny. It's always important, whatever the season, to protect the skin and the lips with sunscreen and lip gloss.

Only one day during the month did it warm up enough for me to ride my bicycle for a short spin out-side. A haughty cold north wind thumbed its nose, numbing my fingers and my toes; my nose ran like a faucet that day from the cold. When the temperature dips down below forty-five degrees, I do not enjoy riding outside, even though I have all the winter gear. Johnny and I often did "basement workouts," a combination of time on our Nordic Track cross-country ski machine and a stationary bike. Through the years we have col-lected various pieces of equipment, often bought on a whim by someone and sold at a discounted price when the piece begins to collect dust. It's definitely advisable to try out a type of work-out machine before purchasing one to be sure it will be convenient and conducive to reg-ular use. My swim coach Carol sold me a little-used treadmill to give Johnny for Christmas. The boys helped me move it into a dark corner of the basement and hide it with a blanket.

We attended "spinning" classes, an intense, forty minute, bicycle-based cardiovascular workout combining cycling techniques with performance visualization. The brainchild of Johnny G., a trainer in California, the craze has caught on in workout clubs across the country. The bike seat and handlebars are adjustable, as is the resistance on the twenty-eight pound flywheel of the specialized Schwinn bicycle. We worked at our own pace, wearing heart monitors to achieve maximum energy output.

Johnny P., a talented cyclist in his own right, led the spinning class on Thursday mornings. We assembled in front of him in two rows, about ten of us in all, women outnumbering men by five to one on most days. As the music started, he had us warm up, bending up and down over the handlebars, gradually increasing the cadence of our feet. "Fast legs, take off... all the way to the end, try not to lock out." The chattering among the group stopped; this period increased my respiration, circulation, and body temperature.

"Now, give it a little tension, get up, don't bounce, don't feel a gap, have a seat, back in the saddle, reach down and get a fast drink." This was the beginning of the conditioning period, geared to increase our cardiovascular fitness, and was intense. My breathing became deeper and my heart was beating faster. Challenging the system is an essential element.

He divided us up into four groups. "Turn the tension up two turns to the right; move your legs at triple speed when it's your turn." These were called "speed bursts."

"*Do it like a lady...*" the music shouted at us.

"Group #1, increase your cadence three-fold, make a complete circle with your feet, keep your upper body still; now stand to the count of six! Have a seat ... now group #2 ...." We went through two of these repetitions, then he increased the number of turnovers to eight, ten, twelve. This went on... and on until we were standing to the count of eighteen.

"Speed up, grab those bars at the end, don't slow down, nice and smooth, use your leverage, take it all the way to the end of the song ...."

"*Do it like a lady...*" I was sweating profusely. I don't know what the guy next to me was imagining; was he doing it "like a lady" too? After a brief respite, we had the music of Limp Bizkit, who sang "Jump up" at just the right time as Johnny P. had us doing "attacks," standing to simulate hills.

"Make sure you have tension on your bike, start climbing with a nice and smooth pedal stroke, focus on technique."

"*Jump up!*" At the very second I thought I could stand no longer, he instructed us to sit to recover.

And then there were "sprints;" our pedal stroke tripled. "Hold it for thirty seconds, let's have 120% effort," he instructed. The end of the song came just at the right time! We grabbed a drink from our caged water bottles and wiped our faces with hand towels. He wandered around the room, making sure that we were all participating (and not in heart failure).

"What's your heart rate?"

"177," responded the fellow next to me, probably twenty years my junior. Mine was 157.

Sweat soaked my t-shirt and my hair, seeping into the red "do-rag" tied around my forehead, protecting my eyes from the burn. It was exhausting... surely making me stronger!

Marcus was our leader on Monday nights. When I first saw his monstrous quads of steel I was suspicious of how he got so strong. I found out.

The music started. "You're on your bike... imagine the road beneath you... ride the white line... ONE GEAR UP. It's 67 degrees and a gentle breeze is blowing... what a day for a ride! ANOTHER GEAR UP... feel the circle, the soles of your feet are separate from your shoes. ONE GEAR UP... heels down... feel the circle... it's all about the circle. ANOTHER GEAR UP... breathe in through your nose, out through your mouth... deep breaths. ANOTHER GEAR UP... give the buns a break (STAND!). DON'T TOUCH THAT DIAL...."

He participated in the class as he gave commands, the music and his voice reaching a huge crescendo after forty minutes. I could close my eyes and see the white line on the road; I was riding the switch-backs of the Alps in the Tour de France! The cool-down included some stretching, on the bike and then off, and allowed the body to readjust gradually to decreased physical demands. The work-outs left me spent, limp, but I recovered quickly and was left with a pleasant sense of fatigue, looking forward to a hearty dinner. These sessions were not competitive. Neither Johnny P. nor Marcus singled out any individual; no comparisons were ever made. Surely my pedal stroke was becoming smoother as my muscles were being primed for better hill climbing.

I started to dream of getting out in the warm sunshine, riding at my own pace, with no one looking over my shoulder and the natural terrain dictating the intensity of my ride! I wanted to roll down a country road to the songs of early spring peepers rather than Limp Bizkit, the smells of blooming lilac instead of body odor, and the sights of delicate green moss sucking up as much chlorophyll as it could before being shadowed by the new leaves on the trees.

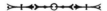

I took time to visit elderly women in a special retirement home just for ladies, believing I was providing holiday cheer to lonely lives. While there I gained one woman's perspective on sons (she had five, Heaven forbid!) and listened in disbelief to another lady's report of a visit by her two sisters who had arrived on their Harley Davidsons. Wise advice on living with boys was assimilated in my brain, and the corroboration of the story of the seventy-ish ladies driving up on their motorcycles lent credence to my belief in the capabilities and toughness of women of all ages.

I answered the plea to donate blood to the Red Cross whose volunteers call me regularly because my O-positive blood type is in demand. The dozens of ever-changing questions about sexual partners, illegal drug use, and where one has traveled always make me wonder how the blood supply can be safe. The volunteer must have wondered what made my lips curl up in a grin as I filled out my questionnaire. I was recalling the recent reaction of my 82-year-old mother, a true southern lady in a monogamous relationship with my father for more than fifty years, when she went to donate her O-negative blood (the gold standard universal donor) for an uncle undergoing surgery. "Imagine it, Emily, they actually wanted to know if I had taken money or drugs for sex, if I had taken cocaine through my nose and if I had had sex with a male who has had sex, even once (!), with another male ... good grief!"

There was a question about whether I had gotten a tattoo during the previous 12 months... maybe a Higher Being had guided my decision not to go there in Hawaii. During the winter months I was happy to share my blood, the temperature-controlling liquid which courses through my veins and those cells which carry nutrients and wastes to and from all body parts, fight infection and provide clotting. The little red blood cells are crucial in providing oxygen to my muscles and organs so I donated with plenty of time to allow them to rebuild before any important competition.

I ate far more than was reasonable; as a matter of fact, I "pigged out." Some Christmas seasons are worse than others. Maybe there were more of those things I love (caramel cake, eggnog, toffee rich with nuts, ...), maybe the stress contributed to overeating. At any rate, I determined not to get on the scales. A weight gain can be a depressing fact which sparks more eating. I knew that when things were "back to normal" I would lose any pounds gained, as long as I continued my regular exercise routine.

It was about that time that my supply of hormones ran out and that, coincidentally, a new study hit the news showing that women taking hormone replacement therapy (HRT) had more dense breast tissue, making mammogram interpretation more problematic. There were so many obligations pulling at me that I let my prescription slide; I decided to go for a while without the hormones just to see how I would feel. A study of one is not a scientific study, but I was curious.

To tell the truth, after two weeks without the medicine I couldn't tell much difference in my energy level (not like it was in my twenties), the severity of night sweats and insomnia (still annoying), libido (a bit on the low side), weight (the same), or the presence of chin hairs (those offensive stiff little black bristles which issue from Heaven Knows Where and beg plucking). I considered giving up the prescription altogether. The hormone fluctuations of the perimenopausal years in my 40's were by and large over. When I think back to those years, I realize how difficult I must have been to live with - I was temperamental, suspicious, and maybe a bit melancholy. Typically after the early 50's, when a woman becomes menopausal, there is a "leveling out," so to speak, and I was feeling this relief.

My knowledge of women's issues has always been supplemented by reading journals which come in the mail. A new one concerning "Sexual Dysfunction" got my attention. Sexual problems among women of all ages are common and affect the majority of women after menopause. The importance of the sexual health of men has given us Viagra, but women's issues are grossly underestimated. Studies support findings that estrogen replacement results in improved clitoral sensitivity, as well as decreased pain and burning during intercourse. It also relieves vaginal dryness, burning, and urinary frequency and urgency. I knew that without hormone replacement there would be irreversible changes to those tissues in my body. My exercise was great protection for my heart, bones, and even brain, but it certainly wouldn't do much for my skin, eyes, or urogenital parts! I made a date for my annual PAP smear and renewed my prescription for "natural" hormones (made of soybeans and Mexican yams - not the same as sweet potatoes), obtainable at the compounding pharmacy near me. These hormones are standardized, meet federal regulations, and require a prescription. They can be given orally or applied on the skin as a cream or in drops.

As far as over-the-counter herbals and botanical products to relieve the symptoms of menopause are concerned, women are flocking into health food stores and ordering them over the internet. One must realize that, because they are not controlled by the FDA, the makers of these products are not required to prove that their products work, or that they are safe, or what side effects can be expected. There has been little conclusive research done on these products in the U.S., though studies are on the horizon, and more clinicians are becoming knowledgeable. If a woman decides to try these products, she should look for high-quality products - look for labels that include the name of the plant used for treatment, a batch or lot number, an expiration date, and how to contact the manufacturer.

In 2005 we would have results of the Women's Health Initiative (WHI), a large randomized, controlled clinical trial, concerning women and their health, including the benefits and risks of taking hormones for extended periods of time (participants were receiving 0.625 mg. conjugated estrogen - "Premarin" - plus 2.5 mg. medroxyprogesterone acetate - "Provera" - or placebo containing no hormone. See Appendix 5). Hopefully before long there would be estrogens which will target selected organs and tissues, sparing others like the breast and the ovaries. In the meantime, I would probably continue to take a low dose of the prescription hormones made from natural ingredients.

A group of us joined for our annual run around the neighborhood to see the Christmas tree lights in the dark. We met at dusk, donned reflective vests and flashing lights, and jogged along the streets. Afterwards we ate hot soup, drank some wine, and indulged in decadent desserts. Carol had had her mastectomy ten days before; she didn't run but she socialized and enjoyed the company.

My training provided a feeling of control over my life as well as my figure. I had been juggling so many things at once during the holiday season, and so often there is no sense of closure in everyday life. With a short run, a swim, a spinning class, or some time in the gym, I felt that I had accomplished something that day. However, the change from my usual training schedule provided a healthy balance. I was contacted by two women to do some individual counseling in women's health issues and set up appointments. Maybe this would jump-start a career with an alternative to the inflexibility of a nine to five job. The news that I had been selected All-American in my age group in both triathlon and duathlon by Inside Triathlon and was ranked third in the country by USA Triathlon provided a great deal of satisfaction.

John came back from New York four days before Christmas, saying to our surprise that things had gone quite well and that he was strongly considering going back to start another semester in January. With three sons in and out of the house at all hours of the day and night our peace was shattered, even though we relished their presence and reveled in their fun.

Johnny and I created our own "private" church service on Christmas Eve - a Sunday morning run in Percy Warner Park. We listened to the sounds of hooting owls, accompanied over our individual head phones by the choir of Christ Church in Cambridge singing carols with the world's finest organ. In place of donkeys and wisemen, we watched Uta bound mystically after white-tailed deer. The multi-sensory experience, fueled by physical exertion, provided a spiritual awareness which we find difficult to match in a church pew. Christmas morning we built a bonfire in the side yard, fixed Bloody Mary's and cooked on a grill for eighteen family members before exchanging gifts.

Keith and Will readied themselves to start back to school. Part of me wanted all three of them to stay home longer. I wanted to cook more blueberry pancakes and big, hearty dinners, to buy a gallon of milk every day; I wanted to wash and fold their clothes, to learn more about their friends. I cherished the moments and knew that if their lives ended the next day my life had been enriched; I regularly whispered prayers of thanks for them. But part of me longed for the solitude of two-for-the-road, my own choice of music, and no phones ringing at two in the morning.

In addition to suffering ongoing discomfort from the pins in his knee, Will had complained that his wrist was still bothering him from a snowboarding injury sustained before his knee surgery last spring; he had been forced to discontinue riding his bike because his wrist hurt so much. His dad got him down to his office three days before his departure to school for an x-ray which revealed an unhealed fracture. He would need to return in a few weeks for more surgery, which would entail a graft from his hip and twelve weeks in a cast; they decided to take the pins out of his knee and scope it at the same time. His winter quarter would be plagued with the logistics of doing school work with his nondominant hand and accepting the hard realization that he would be unable to return to his chosen sport this year.

How do you console a kid who has poured his young dreams into a sport, hoping to make a career of it, and has been beset by terrible misfortune? I tried to talk about it. He either bottled up his feelings well or he was finding school more interesting than he had expected... and he had a girlfriend (his first real one - more sleepless nights for mom - "please be careful" were my parting words).

New Year's Eve. Son John had headed up east into the eye of the worst snowstorm of the year in an old car. We didn't hear from him for several days, in spite of our urgent pleas to let us know when he got to New York.

Keith had plans which would have him out with friends until noon the next day. Johnny and I celebrated the passing of the first year of the new millennium in "dullsville" to the bursts of neighborhood fireworks. It was the wee hours of the morning when Will crept upstairs. The year came to an end. I was tired when, like clockwork, against my wishes, my mind was awake for the first day of a new year. I headed out for a run; I knew I would feel better afterwards.

Keith and Will left for school. The New Year was a collision of fears of the unknown for my children and my aging parents, wonderful memories, and dreams of the future. Underneath those emotions I felt goose bumps erupt when I thought of the Alabama Powerman in March, the qualifier for the World Championship Duathlon in Rimini, Italy, in the fall, and the Vineman Half Ironman Triathlon in California in July, qualifier for the 2001 World Championship Hawaiian Ironman. Before those, though, there were snowy winter trails to snowshoe under nighttime skies of polished ebony, blanketed with zillions of still and shooting stars, and black-diamond ski slopes to negotiate.

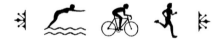

Photos

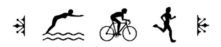

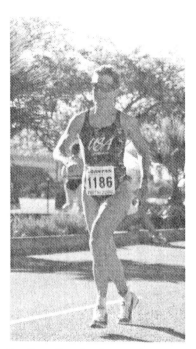

Emily - Perth, Australia 2000

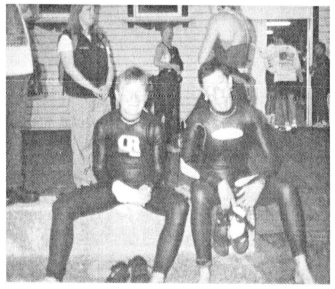

Emily, Ramona Bolander (CA.) - Perth, Australia 2000

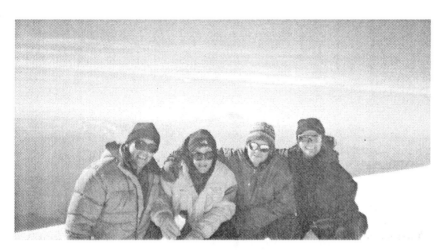

Johnny, Will, Keith, Emily - On top of Mt. Rainier 2000

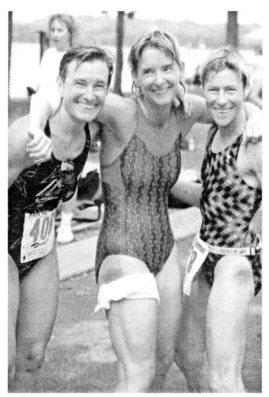

Emily, Liz, and Lyndell. "Road Rash"
Music City Triathlon 2000

167

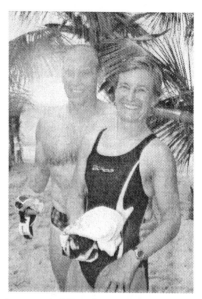

Johnny and Emily - St. Croix 2000

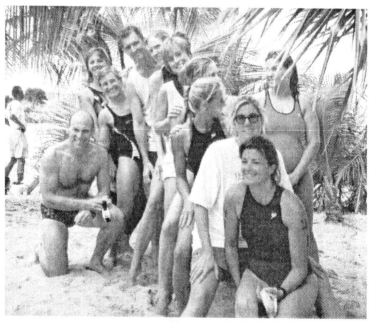

Swim Group - Open Water Swim, St. Croix 2000

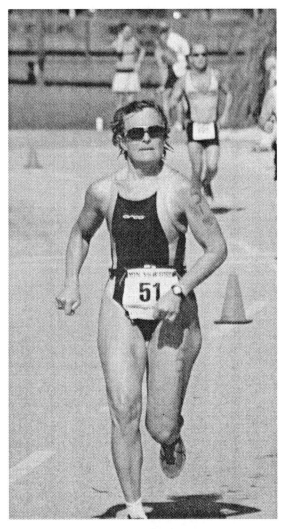

Emily - Tennessee State Championship 2001

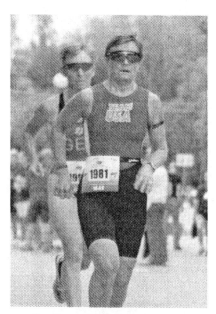

Emily - Rimini, Italy 2001

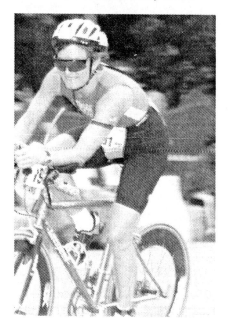

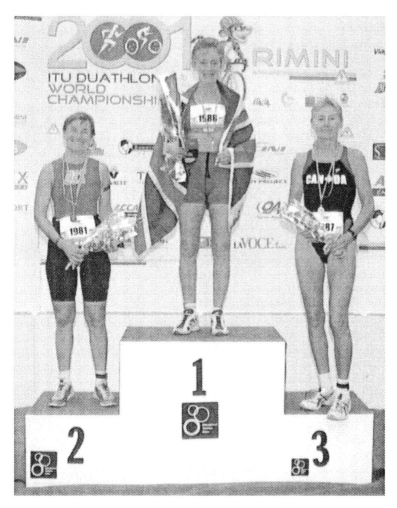

Emily, Elaine, and Linda - Rimini, Italy 2001
Earning the Silver Medal three days after 9/11/01

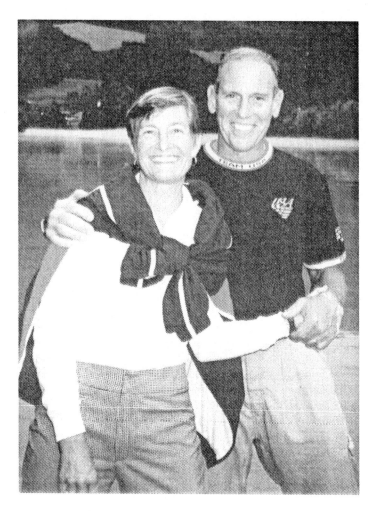

Emily and Johnny - Weyer, Austria 2002

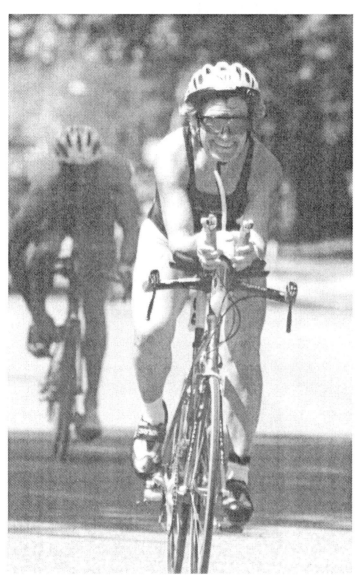

Emily - Maryland "Blackwater - Eagleman" Triathlon
Cambridge, Maryland 2002

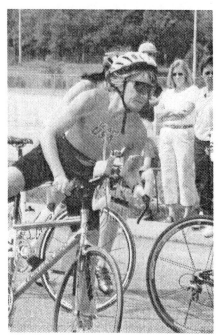

Emily - Powerman Tennessee 2002

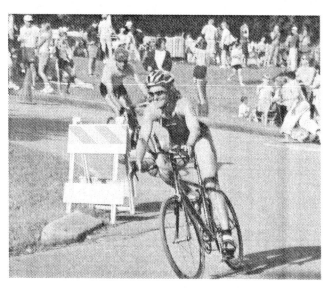

Music City Triathlon 2002

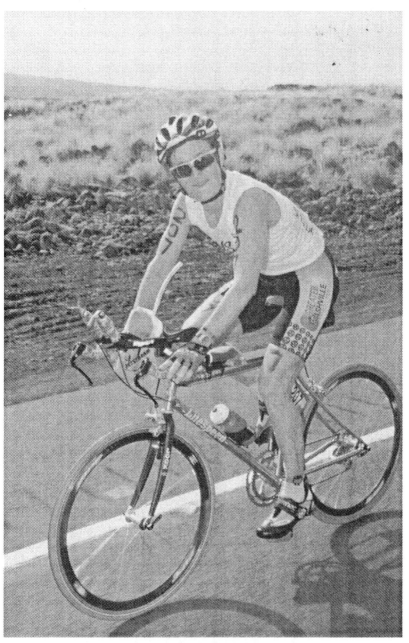

Kona, Hawaii 2002
World Championship Ironman Triathlon

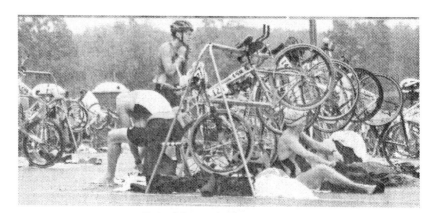

Triathlon transition area

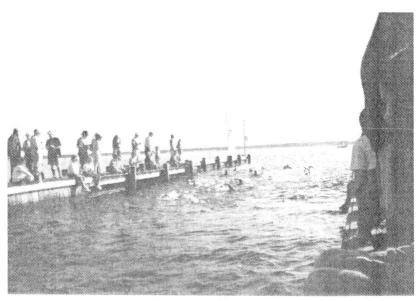

Swimming in the Chesapeake Bay

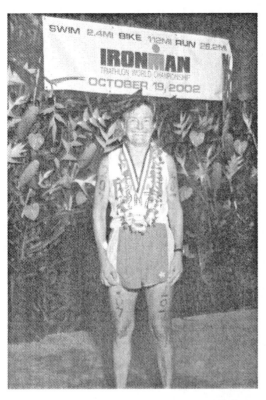

Kona, Hawaii

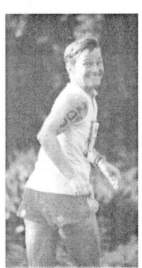

177

2001

*"Let her swim, climb mountain peaks, pilot airplanes, battle
against the elements, take risk, go out for adventure, and she
will not feel before the world .... timidity."*

Simone de Beauvoir

As the new year began, my career as a nurse practitioner was still simmering on the back burner. I kept up my continuing education with meetings and readings and counseled women informally rather than taking on a new nine to five job. I considered an opportunity to help develop a new "Pelvic Floor" clinic. Humor aside, there is a need to help the many women who have urinary frequency and urgency problems after childbirth and may be too embarrassed to seek help. Exercises, biofeedback, and estrogen therapy are common modalities which can prevent the need for surgical intervention. Teaching is important in this new area, and I was interested. But, as I advanced into my new age group of women 55-59 the following September, I wanted to race with quality training; that required a significant commitment of time and energy. During the "off season" of winter, I continued to swim, run, and work out with weights regularly, take short bike rides outside when weather permitted and do spin classes when it didn't. Little did I know how the year would unfold....

My first race of the year was Powerman Alabama,

one of four national qualifiers for the 2001 Short Course World Duathlon Championship in Italy in September. That March morning was sunny but unseasonably cold in the south - in the low thirties. Jo, aged 53, and Ann, aged 56, - arch rivals from many races in the past - were both there to compete. It would be a toss-up: I could beat them when I have a really good race. That day it was hard for everyone racing to decide what to wear; a runner is warmed by the energy expended moving through still air, but the wind chill factor while cycling makes more clothing necessary during that stage.

I started the first ten kilometer (6.2 miles) run with tights, a long-sleeved shirt, and gloves, pulling on an extra jacket before mounting my bike for the sixty kilometer (36 miles) ride. I knew that Jo was a few seconds ahead of me and Ann a few minutes behind as we rushed to start the ride. My legs and hands were comfortable enough, but my toes were numb during the entire bike ride. I struggled with the cold - it distracted me from concentrating on my form and rhythm. The course was very hilly, and I tucked my chin down on my chest, clutched the top tube with my quads, and gritted my teeth as the cold air blew through the vents in my helmet making my eyes tear up as I flew down those hills. That was about as close as I've come to a DNF (Did Not Finish), but that never entered my mind as an option. Johnny and I have always regretted climbing on a bus in the freezing rain in the Boston Marathon of 1980, opting against continuing the race; we sat on that bus for hours with people throwing up all around us and got to the finish line much later than we would have on our own two feet - our DNF was the wrong decision.

Somewhere along that blacktop in Alabama, Ann slipped ahead of both Jo and me (I never saw her). The morning warmed before the final five kilometer run, so

I stripped off some of the clothing before hitting the pavement. I didn't have one of my better races, finishing in three hours and forty-one minutes, five minutes behind Jo, who beat me even after changing a flat tire - she should join those in the pit crews at Indianapolis - but my second place finish (in both the 50-54 and the 55-59 age groups) was good enough for a spot on the USA team for the fall event. By then I would have moved into the older age group. Ann beat both Jo and me with a time of three hours and thirty-three minutes ... and quite a few other women behind us. I had done this exact course the year before in three hours and twenty minutes (we all have some good days - and some better days)!

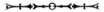

Johnny and I spent the months of late spring and early summer concentrating on open-water swims and longer training runs and rides, preparing for our trip to the Vineman Half Ironman Race in California in July. He was entered as a competitor, too, which made our training compatible. Uta was our constant companion when we ran, as long as it wasn't too hot for her. Whether we chose the trails or roads in the park (where there aren't many cars), she didn't care; unlike us, distracted by watching for rocks and roots lest we trip and sprain an ankle, Uta didn't miss a thing. She sprinted off into the woods or up a steep hill, at the slightest sound or sight which interested her, rarely staying with us, but coming back just in time not to get lost. One day, as we were finishing an hour on the roads in the park, I noticed that she was right between us, trotting like a quarter-horse. I lowered my head to see that she was proudly carrying in her mouth a large motionless squirrel, its thick bushy tail hanging down. We'll never know if she actually caught it, or simply took the spoils, but it was her trophy that day.

Before the trip to California I competed in two other smaller events, placing second woman overall in the Murfreesboro Biathlon with about eighty entrants, running hard against my buddies Lyndell and Liz - both of whom were suffering minor injuries at the time. In its nineteenth year, this was one of the first events in the region combining cycling and running, the competition now called duathlon.

In June, I returned to Chattanooga for the Tennessee State Championship Triathlon. I had a good race, swimming and running strongly and averaging twenty one and a half miles per hour on the bike; when I collected my award for first woman over fifty, the announcer said, "I think we need to check this lady's birth certificate!" I found a good price on some new "race wheels" - more aerodynamic though heavier than my present wheels - at the race expo, where many vendors show and sell goods. As we ate barbecue following the race, I visited with Susan, a friend from Kentucky with whom I've raced through the years. She is in her sixties and has won many national and world championships. We decided to room together over Labor Day weekend in Coeur d'Alene, Idaho, site of one of the two qualifiers for the 2002 World Championship Triathlon in Cancun, Mexico. The other qualifying race would be held in June of 2002 in Lake Placid, New York. We had both heard horror stories of the race held there the previous June: the lake had been extremely cold due to a late spring snow thaw, and many competitors had become hypothermic after the swim. We decided that it would be a good idea to go to Idaho in early September if at all possible....

Johnny and I joined the "3-R's" and Gail, Mary Ann, and Melissa, as well as several other Nashvillians, for the July trip to do the Vineman Half Ironman Triathlon in California. Judy, who swims in my masters group, and Melissa were doing their first race of this distance. We were all planning some fun on the west coast after the race to explore the area and sample wines from the vineyards. I knew that an Ironman qualification was a long shot for me since many new "young bucks" would be there for the event - women just moving into the 50-54 age group.

The application had promised a wetsuit swim in the Russian River, cooled by the spring snowmelt from the mountains. Ray had raced there before and reported that the bicycle and run courses would be "rolling" - not too daunting for those of us who train in the big hills of middle Tennessee. We flew into San Francisco two days prior to the race and drove up the coast to the village of Guerneville, one block from the race start on the banks of the river, to our little motel nestled among giant sequoias. The parking lot provided a great staging area for us to unpack and assemble our bikes and pump up the tires.

The race expo and pre-race meeting were held among the vines of the Kendall Jackson Winery. One of the first announcements made by the race director was that the water in the river was much lower than usual - you could supposedly stand up in it - and was warmer than the seventy-eight degree temperature cut-off to make wetsuits legal. You could hear the disappointment move through the crowd; some even elected not to do the race. With over 2000 participants, my wave would begin shortly after 8:00 a.m., and Johnny's wave (all men over fifty-five) were given gray swim caps and would not even start their race until after 9:30 in the morning! Such a late start would put them out on the sunny course well into the heat of the afternoon. That worried us both.

The group from Nashville made final preparations and had plenty of good carbohydrates and protein the afternoon and evening before the race, hydrating with plenty of liquids... resisting the temptation of anything fermented until after the race! We walked down to see the race site, stood on the bridge above the river and looked at the buoys marking the course, and then stuck our feet in the river - we all agreed that this water was cold enough for wetsuits. But the officials had made their decision; there would be no change to that.

The swim start was not on the beach, but actually in the river. With wild music blasting over the loud speakers, we were herded down to enter the water five minutes before the bullhorn would start our group; we waded in, green swim caps on our heads and goggles covering our eyes, ready to go. Maybe some of the men were tall enough to touch the bottom of the river, but most of us women were too short and thus had to tread water while we jostled for position waiting for the start. There were a few tires floating on the surface of the river, anchored to the bottom, if one could grab a hold; I could feel the goose bumps pop up on my arms and legs as my heart rate increased. As soon as the previously started group was out of sight, the horn was blown, and the temporarily calm water was once again choppy. I tried to swim a "tangent" to make the shortest distance along the snaking river. The swim course was actually longer than the promised 1.2 miles - which one never discovers until after the race when everyone compares his elapsed time in the water. I looked at my watch with disappointment as I came up to the beach to quickly towel off, put on sunglasses, snap the helmet strap, pull on socks and shoes, and remove my bike from the rack. Gail and Mary Ann were cheering and snapping pictures.

I hurriedly clomped through the sand in my bike shoes to reach the pavement where the bike course began, dodging several people falling one way or the other as we all desperately tried to get going up the steep little hill climbing out of the transition zone - I had made sure to put the gears in the lowest possible position early that morning. The bicycle route wound through luscious acres of green vineyards, rolling through small towns just as Ray had promised. There were a few challenging hills - I'll long remember climbing the grueling "Chalk Hill," actually steep enough for some riders to get off and walk up - but the sights and smells were largely 56 miles of light breezes and musky harvest.

I stayed aerodynamic, nibbled the pieces of Powerbar I had stuck to the top tube of my bike, and drank all of my Powerade, passing many people and feeling good. With so many riders out on the course together, I paid particularly close attention to the rules and regulations of the cycling leg of the race. Officials cruise the roads watching for violations; behind the driver of the motorcycle sits someone with a clipboard and pen. They don't tell you at the time if you are in violation, but if the pen touches the paper, a rider hopes it is not his or her number being recorded. Penalties are posted after the race is over. There is a regulation that the helmet chin strap must be buckled whenever you are touching your bicycle, a rule which requires riders to pass others only on the left, and another prohibits taking any unauthorized assistance in food, drink, or bike parts (if you break down or have a flat tire you must be prepared on your own or accept help only from race officials) - these rules are fairly obvious and easy to follow. Even the drafting regulation has become second nature; a drafting zone surrounding each bike is defined. A competitor who enters this zone to pass must either move past the other cyclist within fifteen seconds or fall back. Years ago I had been penalized for a "position" violation. "Charlie," a head referee at a lot of the high-profile races, was someone I came to know at the Gulf Coast Half Ironman Triathlon. When I saw my name posted at the end of that race, I went to Charlie to find out what I had done wrong. He said that I had stayed out too far in the road, potentially "blocking" other riders from passing me (there had been no such riders that I could remember during that part of the race that day). I protested. My rationale had been that I was avoiding a string of potholes in the asphalt along the right edge of the pavement. Charlie had no mercy. The five minute penalty had not cost me a place in that race, but it certainly might in many races, including the Vineman!

I was not exactly sure who my competitors were as I rode in the crowd that day, but I did know that Jo from the Alabama race was there (I had visited with her earlier in the morning). She must have come out of the water before me; I caught her at about mile twenty on the bike, and we played leapfrog during the rest of the ride. We came into the school grounds used for the bike-to-run transition within five seconds of one another. I sat on the ground to change from bike to running shoes, and I must admit that I stayed a little longer sitting on the grass to "pee," my swimsuit wet from sweat anyway! I splashed a cup of water over my front as I ran out.

The day had turned warm, and the miles went from flat to hilly - Ray later admitted that the course had been changed since he had done the race. I saw my younger friends who had started the race in earlier heats than mine, some looking fresher than others, as they were running back to the finish of the 13.1 miles. Shade was sparse on the out-and-back course which circled through the grounds of the LaCrema Winery at the turn-around. I saw Johnny as he was heading out, and I was only three or so miles from the finish. By then it was about one o'clock in the afternoon with the sun high in the sky. He could tell by the look on my face that I was in the throes of hurting, but we came together at the center of the narrow country rode for a high-five and a smile. I worried that he had so much further to run in the heat.

As the finish line approached, I came around the final corner to the shouts of the crowd. With only 0.2 of a mile left, two women approached from behind. I knew Janis from Texas - she had beaten me for the Ironman slot at Memphis-in-May several years ago; she whispered, "Come on, Emily, don't let her go by." Janis was already 55, but I didn't know the other woman - she had my age letter marked on her leg. I picked up my pace, and the three of us raced. I saw Rob on the sidelines and heard him yell, "Go, Emily, run, run, run...!" I should have held back, let them get a little ahead, and started my sprint closer to the finish line; I challenged too soon. They both crossed seconds ahead of me. Regardless of the outcome, it was all I could do to run over the finish line without collapsing.

Realizing that I was about to faint, Mary Ann walked me to the medical area - the first time I've ever had to take advantage of that service. My feet and leg muscles were cramping all the way up and down, sending me into contortions of pain. I took ice packs and cold drinks, but declined the IV. After about twenty minutes on a cot in the cool gymnasium, I felt better and went out to wait for the others at the finish line. Everyone finished. Rob had a terrific race; Ray, Rusty, Melissa, and Judy started telling their stories. Somehow I missed Johnny crossing the finish line; I found him in the massage tent enjoying the healing touch of the therapists on duty - he had finished in good form. None of us had been penalized. I discovered that I had clocked the fastest bike split among the twenty women in my age group, placing sixth in a time of five hours and thirty-five minutes among the 50-54 women. We enjoyed much camaraderie during the hours and days after our efforts, eating wonderful rich food and tasting chardonnays, chenin-blancs, cabernets, and merlots.

>─┼─◆>─O─<◆─┼─<

Later in the month I had a chance to do some mountain biking and hiking in Colorado. A group ride up a dirt road to take in the glorious vistas ended unfortunately with me barreling around a curve too fast on the ride down and losing traction in the gravel. My weight was not properly distributed, the rear wheel skidded out, and I slid on my side in the dirt for what seemed an eternity. I had a bad case of "road rash" and my ego was bruised, to be sure, but no stitches were necessary; I expanded my knowledge of wound care. As the Toyota folks say, "Scars are tattoos with better stories."

One morning at daybreak a group of us bumped along in cars along a dusty gravel road to a trailhead, where we parked and started hiking through a dark green forest beneath cathedral-shaped mountains wrapped in a blanket of blue. The six adults and two dogs first approached Mt. Shavano, one of fifty-plus mountains over 14,000 feet in the state. The official trail was being rerouted, so our fearless leader had us climbing over boulders the size of Volkswagens to attain the summit by early afternoon. Neither Uta nor I was altitude-acclimatized, but our endurance training bolstered our efforts. After a brief rest on the top of Shavano at 14,229 feet, with high winds yanking at the snacks in our gloved hands, we ventured more than a mile further along a sharp saddle to the top of Mt.Tabequashe, a shade shorter at 14,155 feet. Just as the final rays of sunlight sank behind the mountain peaks, we made it back down to the parking lot. We were out of water. Uta was dragging from the day's effort, and my right big toe was bruised from jamming the tip of my boot (I lost that toenail a few months later - not an uncommon occurrence after running a marathon). It took several days of rest for Uta and I to recover. I can't speak for her, but I know I came away with a renewed appreciation for my universe. Never mind that mountain biking and hiking can increase my leg strength, flexibility, and coordination. I felt humbled, yet empowered in the midst of such bold surroundings.

I intensified my training during August, the month before the national championships, adding a weekly session of speed work at the high school track. My friend Lyndell's husband Richard, who has records for his age in various distances in road races, suggested that I do some quarter miles at "race pace." I really didn't want to lose any more sprint finishes if at all possible! I did a mile of slow jogging around the track to warm up before beginning the speed laps. I started with six of the quarters the first trip to the track and planned to add two more each time for three more weeks. The late afternoon sessions were hard, made more so by the above-90-degree, humid weather. During my final session, I felt a pain start in my left hip about halfway through the twelve fast laps. I should have used my good sense and either quit or changed directions (I was running counter-clockwise, and there was no one else there that day). But no, I was determined to complete the plan. I limped to my car. I was no better the next day, despite the ibuprofen, and diagnosed my own problem as an inflamed periformis muscle (or could I have the symptoms of arthritis?) - I had had this same problem the year before. I got in to see the physical therapist Marcus, who validated the periformis diagnosis and did some intense pressure-point work on the hip and electrical stimulation with heat for three days in a row - it was only four days until the trip to Idaho!

People frequently ask me if my running hasn't injured my knees. It is a myth that running causes osteoarthritis, the most common of about 100 kinds of arthritis and a potential burgeoning epidemic among the aging baby-boomers. New studies show that runners are at no greater risk than non-runners, but that athletic injuries and/or congenital mal-alignment may contribute to the disease. Current medical opinion is that the cause of the wearing away of the cartilage in the joints is multi-factorial, with biochemical as well as genetic and mechanical origins; being overweight certainly exacerbates the symptoms. The most susceptible joints are the knees, back, and thumbs. Exercise actually strengthens the muscles and tendons which support these joints and keeps the body's lubricating water flowing; stretching increases range of motion, slowing degeneration of joints through greater flexibility. As for nutritional supplements, I have added a 1500 mg dose of glucosamine to my daily regimen. Though results are conjectural at this time, with scientific evidence pending, significant personal anecdotes support the position that the glucosamine can help reduce pain in joints by building up the joint surface (studies of other supplements are not as convincing).

>-+-4>-+-O-+-<+-+-<

Will and Keith had made their trip to Scotland and Ireland, hitchhiking the byways and illicitly finding jobs abroad to pay for a spot to pitch their tent. They hiked the highlands by day and explored music-filled pubs and dangerous streets in northern Ireland by night.

His surgery behind him, Will was off to the northwest for a semester of school and his renewed pursuit of a career in snowboarding (glucosamine packed), while John elected to postpone higher education again, as he worked in a stained glass studio in Brooklyn. Keith's dream of bigger mountains was fulfilled with acceptance to a semester abroad in Nepal, studying the history and society of the global culture, as well as climbing in the Himalayas. His trip preparation involved a long list of items, which he checked off one by one. He got the required immunizations and visas, and I called to determine if his health insurance was adequate for foreign travel.

"I want to be sure that my son is covered for emergency evacuation... and repatriation of remains," I told the agent. I was reading verbatim the information supplied in the literature sent to us; a period of silence followed.

"Can you hold for a moment while I talk to my supervisor?" she asked. I waited. She returned to the phone with another question, "Do you mean... reincarnation?" I tried really hard not to laugh, thinking of the new religions Keith would be studying, but gradually broke into uncontrollable giggles; the agent joined me, and we both laughed to the point of tears.

"I don't want to talk about death, so I used the words from the booklet, but you know what I mean," I explained. We got that detail worked out. They were off again... at least for a while!

Before leaving, they put a leather bracelet, tanned in Ireland, around my wrist; it was secured with a thin leather shoelace tied in a square knot, the ends trimmed and then glued for permanence. I didn't anticipate keeping the bracelet on for more than a couple of days, but it became comfortable, and I found that it brought me luck in the two most important races of the year, the National Championship Triathlon in Coeur d'Alene and the World Championship Duathlon in Italy.

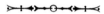

The hip no longer bothering me, I was ready for the trip. As I approached the gate for my connecting flight in Denver, I saw Heidi and Rita, two friends from previous races; they were heading out to do the "nationals" in Idaho, too. While we waited, we caught up on each other's lives since we had been together in Perth, Australia. They had hiked Colorado mountains with mutual friends during the intervening year, and Heidi had recently competed in the Long Course World Championship Triathlon (Ironman distances) in Finland.

My suitcase made the flight into Spokane, Washington, but my bicycle box didn't; there were several other athletes who had the same misfortune. Assured by the airline that they would bring our vital equipment to us as soon as it arrived, we caught the shuttle for the forty-minute ride from Spokane into Coeur d'Alene, where we converged with many more athletes on the host hotel in a quaint little town of the banks of a pristine lake surrounded by mountains. Luckily, my bike followed me several hours later on the next flight. Susan had arrived a day earlier from Kentucky and had already checked into our room.

We had a third person sharing our room - a young woman whom Susan coached on the swim team at the University of Kentucky. Elizabeth had done only three races and was a promising star, having placed in the top three women in each race she had entered. It was like a big slumber party of adults. The room was crammed with three bicycles and many pairs of running shoes, as well as hair dryers and snacks. We lay on our beds in the dark, talking of past events, as well as relationships and children, and gave Elizabeth advice on the finer points of these big triathlons.

During the first two days, we assembled our bikes, went for short rides, tested the cold lake water in our wetsuits, and ate good food. We drove the bike course in a car, which was a good thing, because the course had several steep hills and sharp turns. We went to the traditional women's breakfast, where we learned the status of women in our sport. Celeste, also with us at the World Championships at the Gold Coast in Australia in 1991, was helping to set up novice triathlon clinics; she is the Rocky Mountain Regional representative for the Women's Commission and co-chair of the Judy Flannery Memorial Fund, which provides stipends to qualified multi-sport female athletes. We went to see the film "Judy's Time," the documentary about my friend Judy Flannery who had been killed by a car while training on her bicycle, and wept as we watched the award-winning film made by her daughter Erin. It was wonderful to see Erin again - she had been on the Australian trip with us in 1991 to cheer for her mom - and meet her precious two-year-old daughter named Judy.

The exposition was huge, providing an opportunity to see new clothing and equipment and taste new energy bars. As I gave my race number to enter the expo, I learned that the black number on my calf indicating my age group would be circled, indicating to television crews that I would be highlighted. That was a bit intimidating, though exciting!

The race itself went like clockwork for me - with a few minor hitches: the water was cold and rough, causing some choking; there were not enough buoys, and I swam off course, resulting in a disappointing swim time. But I caught and passed Rita and Ramona (who had beaten me by only seconds in Perth) during the first four miles on the bike. Even though I had seen the course and was aware of one particular sharp turn followed by a steep hill, I shifted my gears too enthusiastically right before the turn and popped the chain off. Sometimes you can pull the chain back on with your foot, but that didn't work for me that day. Luckily, I had enough time to shift the gears down and get the chain back on without having to get off my bike. There was a long hill, climbing over 1,000 feet on a narrow, winding road over more than a mile, and a steep descent ending in a dead end. Hay bales lined the corner in case an out-of-control cyclist were to miss the turn!

The run was two laps of mostly flat road, with lots of supporters yelling and taking pictures. I passed Ann (who had beaten me in Alabama in March) and had a strong finish. Many of us hung out, visited, and waited for the younger finishers who had started after us. Elizabeth came across the finish line and dissolved into tears. She had had a bad swim, and her feet had been numb on the bike and the run; she had really wanted to qualify for Worlds in Cancun and was sure she hadn't. Susan and I bolstered her, assuring her that we, too, have had less-than-perfect races, and that experience has helped us take these disappointments in stride. Awards were given in each's age group on that race day, and six qualifying slots for Cancun were awarded, based on one's age at the time of the race more than a year off. I placed sixth in 50-54, receiving one of Tim's special sculptured metal awards, and second in my new age group, so, either way you looked at it, my mission was accomplished. Unfortunately, there was no time to relax after the race in the beautiful resort, and I tackled the task of packing up for the early morning flight the next morning. As I said good-bye to friends, some of whom would plan a trip the following June to Lake Placid, I was happy I could skip that one!

>--+--+>--O--<+--+--<

I had less than two weeks before the event in Italy, unarguably the most important of the year for me. I hated the fact that I had to unpack and reassemble my bicycle for such a short time, but I knew that there were training rides which I needed to take to maintain my fitness level on the bike. Johnny and many friends competed in the local Music City Triathlon during the weekend I was home, but I "worked" the race, numbering arms and legs with markers before the start on a rainy morning, directing cyclists on the course, and cheering participants; I needed to be "tapering" at that time - still training, but not racing.

On the afternoon of September 10th, Johnny and I boarded an American Airlines jet to Dallas, where we joined about twenty other members of the USA team headed for the World Championship Short Course Duathlon in Italy. Our layover was just long enough to spot some familiar faces before getting situated for the overseas leg of the trip. We passed beneath the setting sun on its journey west as our eastbound flight took us into the twilight through clear, peaceful skies on a trajectory arching up over Pennsylvania, New York, and then the dark waters of the northern Atlantic Ocean. We skipped the movie, covered our laps with blankets, plugged our ears, and pulled on eyeshades to encourage sleep. A farewell thought was never given to the page we tore from the calendar - the last day of innocent, carefree air travel.

A cup of thick espresso after landing at the Brussels airport the following morning revived us long enough to allow us to find our gate for the connecting flight into Bologna, Italy. Still more team members joined us for that final flight on a smaller plane - a plane not big enough for all the bicycles. Unfortunately, about ten of us arrived in Bologna without them; I was one of the unlucky ones! There was much confusion, mainly because the language barrier was huge. None of us spoke Italian, and the workers in the small airport knew little English, so we resorted to hand signals and charts, for which the pictures just didn't seem adequate. Somewhat assured that the bikes would be on the next flight out of Brussels and would follow us soon after, we boarded two large buses for Rimini. Heads bobbed up and down, as we tried to stay awake to appreciate the lush vineyards and orchards and red-roofed stucco houses in the picturesque countryside.

The small town of Rimini, on the Adriatic Sea, hosts tourists from all over Europe; its shady, cobbled streets are lined with shops and cafes, and its beaches invite relaxation. We checked into our hotel and investigated our room, with its ample balcony overlooking the pool below and the wide beach beyond. We quickly unpacked our suitcases and put clothes in drawers while we had the energy. While tackling that chore, Johnny instinctively grabbed the remote and flipped on the television; it is fun to watch how foreign countries handle their entertainment and news. We casually noticed that President Bush's trip to speak to some children in a Florida school was being covered. I looked up from stacking tee-shirts in a drawer just in time to see an aide approach the President from the side and whisper something in his ear. Bush turned his head ever so slightly to the message - a quizzical look, the knitted furrows and curled lip we've seen a hundred times. The report was in Italian.

"Please turn that off. We didn't come to Italy to watch George Bush," I said to Johnny. It was about three o'clock local time - nine o'clock in the morning Eastern Standard Time. I was hungry and wanted to go into town to get something to eat and to explore. We turned off the TV and left the hotel. Each restaurant had its menu posted outside; the choice of pastas was endless - from orecchiette to angel hair. We chose an establishment and sat down outside under an umbrella to enjoy a glass of wine, a meal, a gentle breeze and the afternoon sun.

Another American approached us as we wandered from window to window after finishing our lunch. "Have you heard what has happened in the United States?" Seeing the blank, negative looks on our faces, he proceeded slowly, not really wanting to impose bad news on another countryman. "A plane has flown into one of the World Trade Center Towers" he said. He didn't have an explanation for the "accident" and didn't know the magnitude, but we decided to head back to the hotel to check on my bike and to look for a television channel for news of this event back home.

My bicycle had made it to the hotel. Little did I know then that if it had been delayed for more than just one flight, I probably would not have gotten it for days, if not weeks, because flights had been grounded all over the western hemisphere immediately after the terrorist strikes. We turned the big blue bike case up on its end to fit it into the tiny elevator for the trip up to our room on the fifth floor. I removed the wide red straps from the box, unlatched the top and began to pull out wheels, helmet, shoes, seat post, bike pump - but I stopped what I was doing as I heard the ghastly breaking news. Scanning the channels, Johnny had found BBC and CNN; we were stunned. I sat down with him on the bed, and we stared in horror at the sickening scenes as the sun set over a foreign sea, creating a glorious red sky, clouds and water absorbing and burying the colors.

For hours we just sat there, watching the news and trying in vain to get through on the telephone lines to the States. Tears and anger welled up as we gradually learned that this deed had probably been perpetrated by terrorists. We eventually went to bed, not knowing for sure that John, who was working in Brooklyn, was OK, or if we knew anyone in the area of the Towers or on the flights that had gone down in Washington and in Pennsylvania. I had nightmarish flashbacks of our delayed information when Will had had his accident while we were in Australia and we had remained clueless for two days....

Still unable to make a phone connection to the United States the next morning, we went across the street to an internet cafe and connected with my sister

Susie, who assured us by e-mail that John and other friends and relatives were fine.

It was then time for Johnny's first scheduled clinic for the athletes. He was volunteering his time to the medical staff for the event again, and I attended the team meeting. We sat in rows of chairs facing the stage and our manager Tim. Ordinarily this group of about a hundred athletes would have been chattering and gossiping about the course, the weather, the rules, but we were strangely quiet and tense; there was hushed talk of some team members who had family and friends missing in the attacks. Tim commenced the meeting with a moment of silence as we thought and prayed for our country and the victims, and then he told us that about thirty of our team members' flights had been grounded, and that they might not make it before the event was to begin on Friday. He asked the group if we wanted to participate in this event at all. One athlete spoke up, "I feel that we will show strength and courage if we compete - we must not let the terrorists win by keeping us from our goals and representing our country to the world." Applause started slowly and grew, until everyone in the room was cheering in unison.

"I met with the race director, and he said that you do not have to race in the American uniform," added Tim. I hadn't even considered that some people might fear being targeted by other terror-wielding individuals; most of us were proudly wearing our USA jackets. The group unanimously agreed that we would race courageously and patriotically in the days to come, wearing the red, white, and blue!

The event was to be staged in nine heats over the course of three days, beginning on Friday morning at nine o'clock with all women over forty. I was happy to be in the first group - I could get my race over and then try to enjoy what was supposed to be a vacation for us. I spent plenty of time during the three days before my race eating al-dente pasta and melt-in-your-mouth gelato of creamy green pistachio and frozen tiramisu in a cone and drinking local wine - as well as bottled water - while Johnny made frequent trips to the makeshift clinic at the hotel to treat various ailments among our team members. We watched a lot of television, as images of swarthy faces and names we couldn't pronounce became emblazoned on our minds.

David, my favorite massage therapist who travels to many of the team events, gave me a pre-race rubdown, and I shopped for gifts at the sports expo. The master list of athletes was not complete - the organization seemed even more haphazard than the year before in France. Tim refused to let us register ourselves and faced the hoards for us; he said that when this event was held in Italy before, competitors showed up from all over the world to register up until race day, so any predictions I might make of my competition were useless.

Our hotel was conveniently located only a block from the race course, which made it appear easy to plan and execute short training runs and rides on the course. The biggest problem was that automobile traffic raged along the road, so, while running on the sidewalk was safe, biking was not safe anywhere! There would be six loops to the bike part of the race, each one a little over four miles. After assembling the bike, I elected to make only one test loop. I was proud that I could handle my own mechanical needs and didn't require the help of the bike mechanic who traveled with the team.

Friday morning dawned cool and gray. Johnny left to collect the medical supplies and go down to the transition area; I spun the wheels of the bike in the hotel room to make sure they weren't rubbing the brake pads, put on my backpack holding all of my gear, and walked the bike down to the city park where the race would begin and end. As I approached the transition area I found Tim; he was putting a black armband around any athlete who wanted to have it, in recognition of our tragedy at home. All Americans seemed to want this symbol, and some competitors from other countries followed suit. After getting my gear arranged, I looked around at the other women - I was especially interested in those with red banded numbers. This method of numbering seemed better than the leg marking (which could easily be covered by tights); each person was to wear a number attached to her back and her front. Women 55-59 had numbers banded in red; there should be no one incognito - if the rules were followed.

When the starting horn blew, about a hundred women bolted; I had placed myself on the second row, knowing that some of the younger women in their forties would probably be faster. Near me were about three others in my age group. This was not a race where I could hold back and hope to catch up later, so I pushed myself to stay with them. The first run was two loops of five kilometers each, offering several turns and an opportunity for spectators to watch at one intersection and turn around to cheer the group coming from another direction; the loud speaker could be heard almost everywhere. The course was flat and fast.

After about fifteen minutes of hard running, I could hear a woman's heavy breathing right behind me; she was drafting off me as we made a turn into the wind along the sea. I became annoyed that she wouldn't back off some. Just as I motioned with my hand for her to give me some space, she stepped on my right heel! Luckily, my shoe didn't come off. She said something, but it didn't sound like "I'm sorry." I decided to slow down briefly, let her go by, and run along beside her. As we picked up the pace, she slowed down a lot; I later learned that she was on the German team and had dropped out.

Out on the bike, the wind blew hard from the south; I tried to stay down and aerodynamic. There have been races where athletes have lost track of the number of loops and have been disqualified. So the trick of peeling off one of five pieces of duct tape after each of the six laps worked well - after the last piece is gone, you know you're on your last lap! Johnny cheered and snapped pictures as I rounded the fountain after each lap. He didn't yell out where he thought I stood; both of us knew that such conjectures had proven false in the past! Americans who would be racing in other heats were also out cheering. I saw one woman in my age group in the other lane ahead of me, but I was uncertain of who else might be there. I never felt I was riding particularly well, battling the wind and feeling a drag when I passed over the timing mat at each turnaround. Anne, an American in the 50-54 year old group passed me during the fourth lap (I had beaten her in Powerman Alabama and in Coeur d'Alene - either she was having a great day or I was not having a particularly good one), but I never saw a red-bordered number go by.

I finally rode into transition, sat down on the towel next to my bike, and yanked off my biking shoes to pull on my racing flats for the final five kilometer run; a tight cramp grabbed my calf. I slowed my movements a bit and told myself to "get over it" as I jumped up. I tackled the final five kilometer run and felt strong as I began to hear the voice over the loud speaker announce the names and countries of those who were finishing.

As I ran, I heard her announce that at noon there would be three minutes of silence around the world, remembering the lives lost in the events of the previous Tuesday. I was about three blocks from the finish when the crowds stopped their shouting and became perfectly quiet and still; I briefly wondered if I should stop, in respect, but knew in my heart that that would not be expected of me. I rounded the final corner in a sprint to the finish, uncertain who might be behind, to spectators observing complete and total silence. What a bizarre finish line!

Waiting there was Elaine from Britain, who hugged me and whispered that I had placed second, two minutes behind her. Soon the cheering resumed, and in two more minutes, Linda from Canada came in, taking the bronze in our age group. Johnny was taking pictures, allowed in the restricted area because of his medical pass. As we were ushered to the podium, someone offered me an American flag to hold, along with the bouquet of flowers presented by the governor of Rimini. My eyes welled with tears. To have earned a silver medal for my country in a week of such tragedy brought strong emotions.

After visiting with other racers and having refreshments, I made my way back to the hotel room for a hot shower. As I leaned the bike against the wall, I spun the wheel one more time. It stopped against the brake pad before even one revolution! I had run my fastest run splits in many years, but I'll forever wonder what could have been possible if I had let the bike mechanic take a look at my bike....

During the remaining days and races, the weather deteriorated. There were thunderstorms and bike wrecks, but we supported our friends, and the Americans persevered. At the official award ceremony on Sunday night, our country collected the most number of medals of all the countries, even though about twenty of our team members had never made it to Italy.

We had planned to spend two days in Rome after the race, along with about thirty other team members. We stuck with that plan, knowing that it would be impossible, as well as unnecessary, to attempt to get home sooner, even though we felt like expatriates in our distant suffering for our land. Wandering through ancient Roman ruins under the Italian sun and studying gorgeous mosaics on floors and glass in the windows of cathedrals and museums reminded us of the relative youth of our homeland, and we appreciated the kindness of the world outside of America.

Security was lengthy and tight on the flight home. As we made a hurried connection in Dallas, my bike box was opened, not only to search for weapons and/or contraband, but to disinfect the wheels in case of possible contamination by hoof and mouth disease. I brought home with me a deep gratitude that I live in a country where women are allowed to study, to work, and to express ourselves in a myriad of ways, a silver medal, and five extra pounds. The only thing I didn't care to keep and protect was the five pounds!

>−¦ ◆⟩·◯·⟨◆·¦−◅

My last race of the year, the Race for the Cure, was not run for me but for Adrienne, Barbara, Carol's mom Rita, Florence, Judy, Virpi, Gwynn, Lois, Emily, Molly, and Betsy, all friends whose lives have been touched by breast cancer. The Susan G. Komen Breast Cancer Foundation sponsors this event, which began as a local race for women-only, with only 125 runners ten years ago, to an event with almost 8,000 men and women. The largest series of 5k runs/fitness walks in the world, it is now held in more than 100 cities in this country and in three foreign countries with more than 1.3 million participants. The funds raised are dedicated to education and research on breast cancer causes, treatment, and the search for a cure. The race falls at the end of an entire month of luncheons and seminars geared to increasing awareness of the importance of early detection of breast cancer.

The day of the race, I proclaimed my friends' names on a card pinned to the back of my shirt for all to see, and the knowledge of their courage was carried in my heart every step of the way. Personal stories and motivations were shared on a lovely fall morning. It was appropriate that no age group awards were given; it didn't matter how fast or slowly one ran that day - just being there in the moment was what mattered.

Coincidentally, that fall new observational studies were surfacing, making the issue of the health benefits and risks of hormone replacement therapy (HRT) after menopause much murkier than it had appeared before. Clinical trials were showing an increase in breast cancer, especially lobular tumors which are rarer than the ductal ones and are harder to detect, among long-term hormone users (greater than five years). Risk was greater among women on estrogen and progestin (that's me!) than in those on estrogen alone. These increased risks appeared to drop back to average within about five years after a woman stops the hormones. The studies intimated that, though hormones do help prevent bone thinning, they may not prevent bone fractures (calcium, vitamin D and the new class of "designer estrogens" do more in this regard).

Perhaps the most troubling were the studies showing that HRT does not prevent heart disease (and may actually increase the risk of strokes and blood clots in some healthy women). The belief that we could extend the premenopausal protection of our cardiovascular system conferred by our hormones beyond menopause with replacement therapy was erased. (In May, 2002, after a mean of 5.2 years of follow-up, the researchers of the Women's Health Initiative - WHI - stopped the hormonal arm of the study when it became clear that the Premarin/Provera therapy increased the risk of heart attack, breast cancer and blood clots and that benefits were more subtle than previously thought. The FDA presently recommends that if HRT is used to relieve menopausal symptoms, it be used at the lowest dose that works and for the shortest possible length or time. See Appendix 5. See more at www.4woman.gov.)

We were back to the drawing board and the cold hard truth - that heart disease is the number one killer of women, striking down more women than all cancers combined. And, unlike breast cancer, we do have a handle on major causes of the disease: smoking, diabetes, high blood pressure, high cholesterol levels, excess weight and physical inactivity.

Quality of life enhancements for women on HRT, such as the reduction in the severity of hot flashes, may continue to make it worthwhile for the first few years after the onset of menopause, but the choice is certainly not as clear-cut. All of this serves to underscore the value of a healthy lifestyle in disease prevention and longevity, as well as quality of life. I would venture to say that exercise may play perhaps the most important role!

>─┤◆〉─〇─〈◆├─◁

One more year's calendar was complete. Like colorful butterflies molting from caterpillars into adulthood, the boys flittered in and out. John left New York ("I don't relish getting on the subway or crossing the bridges"), sold everything, and bought a motorcycle - Will called him "Easy Rider." Will became strong from long distance cycling and returned to the slopes to pursue his dream of being a professional snowboarder. Keith made it safely back from the Himalayas, loaded with stories and other gifts, returned to school to finish his final two semesters, and found new love.

I planned to keep running, biking, swimming, strength training, and climbing mountains for myself and for other women. For fear of sounding self-affirming, I hoped not to prove my unique worth to the world by my competition, but to share with other women, especially those also in their years of changing bodies and responsibilities, the bone-deep satisfaction which comes from stretching physical limits and setting new goals. I had done things which made me feel the blessings of my life. I had felt the energy of representing my country in foreign lands, sharing a universal joy and passion with other women, and had worn the red, white, and blue on the medalists' podium.

All women can let go of the nuisances and problems of life and allow themselves to tap into the abilities of their bodies, changing random attempts at healthy living into habits, setting goals and reaping heretofore unknown rewards from lives of self-discipline and discovery. I, like every woman, whether young, perimenopausal or postmenopausal, am a work in progress. I don't plan to be doing 720's on a snowboard park halfpipe; but who knows, some year soon Johnny and I might take to the Trail!

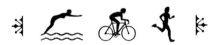

Afterword

>─┼─◆>──O──◁◆─┼─◁

2002 was a year of extremes - there were moments of loss and sadness, fear and fright, accomplishment and ecstasy. In the early spring Johnny and I both qualified to represent the USA for the Long Course Duathlon World Championship to be held in Weyer, Austria, in August. I won the Masters' Division at Powerman Tennessee, one of two qualifying races, and he placed eighth in his age group (the selection for the team went eight deep!) He said, "This may be the only time in my life that I will be on an American team - let's go."

The race course in the mountains of Austria sounded very difficult from the first information we received. We studied maps sent on-line from manager Tim and planned training runs and bicycle rides with lots of hills. The Austrian event would be a run-bike-run format, with two 4.7-mile run loops, two 28-mile bike loops, and would finish with running one of the first 4.7 mile loops again. In June, both of us had completed the Blackwater/Eagleman Half-Ironman Triathlon in Maryland, a good test of endurance in the heat, though that course lacked the mountains we would find in Austria. At the Maryland race I won my age group, and a fifteen-year anniversary trip to the Hawaiian Ironman - the Superbowl of the sport - was planned. Only three weeks after that event, I would fly to Cancun for the Short Course World Championship Triathlon. We felt that the race in Austria would be a good tune-up for me.

We were assigned for lodging in Weyer to the Post

Hotel, large by village standards, but family-owned and operated, lending a homey feel. Thick wooden planks lined the floor of the huge dining hall which the team immediately converted into a place to unpack and assemble our bikes and store the big boxes used for transporting them. The days leading up to the event were passed in practice runs on forest footpaths out of the village where the race would begin and bike rides along the Ebbs River, up the hairpin curves into the mountains with a gain of over 1,200 vertical feet, then descending and climbing again through the village of Grossraming before winding back along the river banks into Weyer.

We enjoyed being immersed in the culture and sampled the wide array of Austrian beers. Nashville friends Rob and Melissa were staying with a local family who treated us to champagne around their kitchen table, as we tried to communicate with our minuscule German language skills and their broken English; Heinz drove us to their country home, where he hand fed a family of European deer on a daily basis. The weather in the mountains was unpredictable, often changing hourly from clear blue skies to sudden showers.

The morning of the race was gorgeous, though quite warm. There was a "citizens' event" to begin the day, with all comers competing in a shortened version of the course we would be doing. To allow time for digestion, Johnny and I had an early breakfast and made our final preparations, pumping up our tires and assembling our race drinks and food before taking everything to our mutual transition areas. I threw in a long-sleeved shirt at the last minute, thinking it might prevent an evening chill immediately after the race. We found shade, stretched, and snapped pictures during the morning hours.

As race time approached, spectators gathered shoulder-to-shoulder, several bodies deep behind the restraining tape, balloons bobbing in bunches across the lanes; everyone contributed in one fashion or another to a party mood. At 12:45 the women assembled behind the starting line on the main road in the village. The pro women would start at 1:00, followed three minutes later by the rest of the females. The men's event would begin at 1:15. "I will meet you at the finish line," I said to Johnny, as we kissed good-bye; "please be careful."

Through our twenty-plus years of racing, I would look for him at points where we might overlap on a race course and worry about his safety; he rides with abandon, and my concern was usually about his having a bike wreck. But in recent years, because of his elevated cholesterol and blood pressure, my fears had become more generalized. He had regular check-ups and had been on medication to lower the cholesterol and regulate the blood pressure, but there was little to do about the risk factors of a family history of heart disease and the job stress he experienced. A thalium stress test and fast CT of his heart just months before had shown high calcification but no blockages. He had always exercised for health, and there appeared to be no contraindications now.

The temperature climbed during the morning hours; when the horn was blown, the sky was cloudless. It was hot! Race strategy for most of us was to do the first two run laps at a pace which would not deplete reserves for the tremendous challenge to follow in the mountains. Many competitors, including Johnny, were wearing heart rate monitors. He reported later that his pulse had almost immediately jumped higher than his intended zone.

Within the first hour of the race, the sky suddenly

became dark, and it started to pour. I lost track of the competitors in my age group. At first I reveled in the coolness, and my mind momentarily drifted to dreams of windshield wipers for my sunglasses. But the crashing thunder and jolting lightning bolts nibbled at my confidence and made me begin to question the sanity of cycling in the mountains. As I ran into the transition zone to the cheering of the villagers, freshly committed to mounting my bike, I remembered the long-sleeved shirt and started to tie it around my waist, but heeded the advice from an American on-looker beside the fence who said, "Put it on now or you never will! Go, girl!" The shirt probably saved me from hypothermia.

The storm abated somewhat as I started the first climb. I narrowly warded off muscle cramps in my feet and legs, pushing down and pulling up hard on the pedals, and wished for an easier gear. And then came a dangerous, fast descent over wet roads as I tucked into an aero position and resisted using the brakes. I began to feel a bit better with the completion of the first lap through the cheering crowds in Weyer, cow bells clanging, music blasting, volunteers offering bananas and energy bars. The announcer yelled the country of the competitors as we rode through to begin our second loop on the bike. I definitely felt better; whereas Johnny later said he never got that "second wind."

The final run was complicated by muddy sections on the forest paths, causing competitors to slip and slide, and some were falling. As I approached the finish, I saw Johnny coming out of transition to begin his last run. We both smiled and shared quick words of encouragement; seeing him made me happy. I would finish in about five hours, and I figured he would be maybe forty minutes back. I collected my finisher's shirt, pulled it over my damp torso to ward off a chill, and went to the corner right next to the transition area, gathering with three other Nashvillians to cheer other Americans and wait for Melissa and Johnny to finish.

We waited forty, then fifty minutes, and the time lengthened to an hour. The others left to collect their things as the mountain air cooled. The Austrians sweeping the route on bicycles said that there was no one else left out on the course; they said to go ask the announcer for information. As I walked away from transition with my bike and bag of wet clothes, Tim approached, "Emily, Johnny is OK, but he has had a myocardial infarction."

At first, I thought Tim was joking (denial on my part). I had seen Johnny smiling only an hour before, with just 4.7 miles left in his race; but the look on Tim's face convinced me otherwise. "The van is waiting there to take you to the hospital in the next village. I'll take care of your and Johnny's things." I dropped everything and ran over to get in the van.

After a thirty minute ride, accompanied by the American team doctor who confirmed that Johnny was stable, I found him in the cardiac intensive care unit, monitors beeping and tubes running in all directions. He was groggy, but told me the details of what had happened: he had not felt well from the beginning - the heat and then the sudden storm had depleted him. He had considered quitting after the first run, and again after the first bike loop, but was energized by all of the spectators along the course - and he kept thinking of that finisher's t-shirt.... Eventually, the generalized fatigue became chest pain that wouldn't go away with walking, and he gave in and hailed a ride to the first-aid tent. His comment that he had muscle cramps, but that maybe they "should check the S-T segment of my EKG" met with quick attention. The test revealed that he was in fact having a heart attack, and an ambulance was summoned. (At that point he was just yards from the corner where I was waiting!)

The trauma doctor in the ambulance offered him the "clot-busting drug" (which is administered in the U.S. only after a patient has arrived at the ER); "Do you know the risks?"

"Yes I do - go ahead and give it to me!" he answered. That fast action, which left him with painful bruising up and down his left arm, may have saved my husband from permanent heart damage. A second dose was given thirty minutes later.

The doctors seemed competent, and the communication was better than I hoped. They assured me that he was stable and that I could return to the hotel to clean up and that they would call me if there was any change. "I'm staying here... in that chair," pointing to the hall outside the ICU. I requested a sheet to pull over my shoulders as I shivered in my sweaty race togs.

Our new Austrian friends brought Melissa to the hospital later that night. She arrived with a bag of clean clothes for us and my bronze medal for my third place finish. She offered to pack up and take our bikes on their flight back home; she would tell the hotel what had happened and that I needed to keep the room another night. The hospital staff, accepting the fact that I was going nowhere, brought me soup, bread and yogurt, directed me to a shower, and provided a cot for the night.

The following day we were transported by ambulance to Linz, a larger city, where a cardiac catheterization was done. The discovery of a narrowing in the right coronary artery resulted in a stent for Johnny. I rented a car and trekked back down to Weyer to retrieve our things from the hotel. The Post was quiet after the departure of all the Americans. The young lady at the desk called her brother because she couldn't speak English. When they understood my explanation that my husband was recovering well after his heart attack, their eyes moistened, and they embraced me. I pulled out my wallet to pay for the extra two nights but they wouldn't hear of taking my money. The room was just as we had left it two days before; our friends had emptied our bike bottles to prevent mold and spread out our wet and dirty race clothes to dry.

There was considerable finagling with the airlines. At first, they claimed to have no coach seats available for a month (we could fly home business-class for $5,000). When I explained, "You don't understand. We didn't choose this; my husband had a heart attack" - there was another reaction.

The female voice said "Goodness! We don't allow anyone to fly for four weeks after a heart attack!"

After numerous desperate calls to the travel agent, we were allowed to fly home (with the doctor's permission) three days after our planned departure. In my private moments during the ordeal, I had decided that the October Ironman trip to Kona and the November Short-Course World Championship Triathlon in Cancun were no longer important to me; they just didn't matter any more.

There were dozens of get-well messages and acts of kindness upon our arrival home. Reactions ranged from "if he had a heart attack, why don't I just keep sitting on my sofa and eating my chips" to "he might be dead if he weren't so fit!"

For follow-up care we decided on a cardiologist who happened to be an ultramarathoner himself; not everyone understands the mentality of those of us who need our exercise endorphins. As the days progressed, Johnny started back to work and became more confident with his recovery (walking, jogging, and biking) and cardiac rehab. I resumed my training, and we decided to stick to my fall schedule.

He was on the pier for the canon start of the Ironman in Kona and on the sand beach for the race in Cancun. We got a new video camera, so that we could watch this when "we're in our eighties." There were moments of doubt and darkness on the lava fields in Hawaii, but the astonishing day ended with me in sixth place. I endured the relentless heat of the blazing sun in Mexico, placing second among the American women in my age group and seventh in the world. I knew I would be all right - because he had promised "I will see you at the finish line."

Our friend Lois lost her battle with cancer, but I could imagine the twinkle in her eye and a hand raised with a high-five as her words rang strongly, "You go, Girl!"

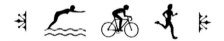

Afterword

Appendix One:
A Suggested Exercise Program for Women

Physical activity has been associated with the prevention and control of many medical conditions (heart disease, hypertension, diabetes, osteoporosis, obesity, and mental health problems). If a woman has no history of heart trouble, chest pain, dizziness, high blood pressure, bone or joint disease, or any other contraindication, she may begin an exercise program which should include something that involves each of the following three basic components. Different portions may be done on alternating days. It is not necessary to "take a day off."

Cardiorespiratory endurance:
Intensity: heart rate should be in the "training zone" - 220 minus her age times 60% to 80% (she should "sweat")
Frequency: 2 to 4 times per week
Duration: 30 to 40 minutes
Brisk walking for short 10-minute periods, as a first stage for untrained, sedentary women; progress to more vigorous levels including running, biking or some form of cycling, or swimming.

Muscular Strength (Resistance) training:
Frequency: 2 to 3 times per week, with a rest day between sessions
Weight lifting, partial sit-ups and other site-specific weight-bearing exercises.

Flexibility:
　　Frequency: daily for 10 to 15 minutes, after "warming up"
　　Stretching exercises which improve the ability to move the joints and use muscles through their full range of motion.

Note: Noncompliance with physical activity programs is typically 50% after the first 6 months and is similar to that seen for other health-related behavioral interventions, such as smoking, substance abuse, and dieting. Having a partner to whom one is accountable increases the chance for success.

Appendix Two:
Body Mass Index (BMI)

Body Mass Index Table (For Women and Men)

1. Read down the first column to locate your height.
2. Read across that row and locate your weight.
3. Read the heading on top of the column - that's your BMI.

Height (inches)	18	19	20	21	22	23	24	25	26	27	28	29	30	31+
58	86	91	96	100	105	110	115	119	124	129	134	138	143	148+
59	89	94	99	104	109	114	119	124	128	133	138	143	148	153+
60	92	97	102	107	112	118	123	128	133	138	143	148	153	158+
61	95	100	106	111	116	122	127	132	137	143	148	153	158	164+
62	98	104	109	115	120	126	131	136	142	147	153	158	164	169+
63	101	107	113	118	124	130	135	141	146	152	158	163	169	175+
64	105	110	116	122	128	134	140	145	151	157	163	169	174	180+
65	108	114	120	126	132	138	144	150	156	162	168	174	180	186+
66	111	118	124	130	136	142	148	155	161	167	173	179	186	192+
67	115	121	127	134	140	146	153	159	166	172	178	185	191	198+
68	118	125	131	138	144	151	158	164	171	177	184	190	197	203+
69	122	128	135	142	149	155	162	169	176	182	189	196	203	209+
70	125	132	139	146	153	160	167	174	181	188	195	202	209	216+
71	129	136	143	150	157	165	172	179	186	193	200	208	215	222+
72	132	140	147	154	162	169	177	184	191	199	206	213	221	228+

BMI under 19: Underweight
BMI 19 to 25: Healthy weight
BMI 26 to 30: Overweight
BMI 31 and over: Obese

Appendix Three:
Recommended Nutritional Supplementation

Vitamin C, 500-1000 milligrams (mg.) per day

Vitamin E, 400 international units (IU) per day

A multivitamin, including folic acid and the other B vitamins, 400 IU Vitamin D, Vitamin K and trace minerals

Calcium, enough to bring the daily total to 1,200-1,500 milligrams (mg.), taking into account dietary calcium, in divided doses (calcium carbonate must be taken with food)

Glucosamine, 1,500 milligrams (mg.) per day

For consideration: Aspirin, 81 milligrams (mg.) per day

Appendix Four:
Recommended Preventative (Diagnostic) Testing After the Onset of Menopause (In addition to, or as part of, an annual head-to-toe "well-woman" examination)

>-+-+>-+O-+<-+-+-<

Screening for genital and cervical disease/cancer:
Pelvic examination: annually
PAP smear: annually, or every 2-3 years with no risk factors, at the discretion of the caregiver

Screening for breast disease/cancer:
Breast self-examination: every month
Breast clinical exam: annually
Mammography: 40 years and older, annually

Screening for bone thinning and osteoporosis:
Dual-energy x-ray absorptiometry (DEXA): onset of menopause and then as needed

Screening for colon cancer:
Digital rectal exam: 40 years and older, annually
Stool blood test: 50 years and older, annually
Sigmoidoscopy or colonoscopy: 50 years and older, every 5 years

Screening for hyperlipidemia (elevated cholesterol), diabetes, hypo- or hyper-thyroidism:
Relevant blood work at recommended intervals

Regular dental and opthomological exams

Appendix 5:
Understanding the Women's Health Initiative (WHI) Study

The combination hormone replacement therapy (HRT) component of the study was not designed to assess the relief of menopausal symptoms, such as hot flashes, night sweats, and vaginal dryness, but to investigate the long-term benefits and risks of estrogen plus progestin therapy, usually prescribed to those women who have not had a hysterectomy. The combination HRT component of the study was discontinued after an average follow-up of 5.2 years because the risks outweighed the benefits. The estrogen-alone arm of the study continues. This study was conducted through the National Institutes of Health (NIH); more can be found at www.4woman.gov.

The chart below shows the increase/decrease in health events per 10,000 women annually for those not taking HRT (placebo) vs. those taking combination HRT.

	10,000 women/year taking placebo	10,000 women/yr taking combination HRT	Difference per year
Breast cancer	30	38	8 more women with breast cancer
Heart attacks	30	37	7 more women with heart attacks
Strokes	21	29	8 more women with strokes
Blood clots	16	34	18 more women with blood clots
Colorectal cancer*	16	10	6 fewer women with colorectal cancer
Hip fractures*	15	10	5 fewer women with hip fractures

* HRT is not indicated for the prevention or treatment of colorectal cancer or hip fractures. See more at www.4woman.gov

Index

Pilates, 45, 88
Pre-race meal, 36-37, 118, 184
Preventative testing, 97, 99, 159, 221
Progesterone, see hormones

R
Road rash, 106, 188
Running with your dog, 88-91, 181-182
Running and walking, 32, 71, 81-83, 137-138

S
Scuba diving, 48, 130
Sharks, 21, 37, 77, 108, 128, 130, 135
Sex after menopause, 132, 160
Side stitch, 106
Sigmoidoscopy, see preventative testing
Spinning, 154
Strength (resistance) training, 33, 148,
   217-218
Stretching and flexibility, 21, 45, 58, 83,
   157, 190, 217-218
Supplements, including vitamins and
   herbals, 76-77, 101, 160-161, 190-191, 205,
   220
Swimming, 53-54, 153-154

T
Tapering, 28, 35, 50, 59
Tattoos, 53, 158, 188
Testosterone, see hormones
Triathlon history, 26-27, 69, 108
Triathlon race rules, 62, 185-186
Title IX, 68

V
Vitamins, see supplements

W
Waist-to-hip ratio (WHR), 30
Wave starts, 37
Wetsuites, 21, 33, 37-38, 53, 106, 183-184
Women's Health Initiative (WHI), 161, 206,
   222
Working out with weights, see strength
   training

Y
Yoga, 45

About The Author

Emily Bruno was a team player in high school, enjoying field hockey, soccer, and basketball. After a distinctly non-athletic college career and early adult life, she became interested in running and later in multisport events as a way of controlling weight and sharing time with her husband, a former college football player and sportsmedicine orthopaedic surgeon. After almost twenty years in the sport, she has completed eleven marathons, two ultra-marathons, numerous road races, duathlons, and triathlons. She has been selected All American several years, earned the silver and bronze medals in the World Championship short- and long-course duathlon and been on the American team in the short-course triathlon in Australia and Cancun; she was ranked first American grand master (over 55) duathlete in 2002. She finished fifth in her age group in the 1987 World Championship Hawaiian Ironman Triathlon and sixth in 2002 and will compete on the American team in the World Championship short-course triathlon in Madiera, Portugal, in 2004.

When her children were teenagers, the author went back to school to earn a master's degree in nursing because of her interest in women's health and nutrition; then worked as a nurse practitioner. She has written articles and spoken on panels about osteoporosis, nutrition, and exercise and enjoys sharing her passion with other women.

The Brunos spend their time in Nashville, Tennessee, and Crested Butte, Colorado.

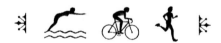

Ordering Additional Copies

To order additional copies of Ironwomen Never Rust, please complete this form and mail with your check or money order to:

> Emily Bruno
> 621 Westview Ave
> Nashville, TN 37205

Your mailing address:

Name: _____

Address: _____

City: _____

State: _____ Zip Code: _____

Telephone: _____

Email Address: _____

Amount you need to enclose:

Send: _____ books at $16.95 US each: _____

Tax at 9.25% *(Tennessee residents only)*: _____

$4.00 S&H for the 1st book: _____

$2.00 S&H for each additional book: _____

Total amount enclosed: _____

You may also order on the internet at:
www.westviewpublishing.com

Printed in the United States
20962LVS00002B/129-228